NUTRITION AND DIET RESEARCH PROGRESS

IRON DEFICIENCY AND ITS COMPLICATIONS

NUTRITION AND DIET RESEARCH PROGRESS

Additional books in this series can be found on Nova's website under the Series tab.

Additional E-books in this series can be found on Nova's website under the E-book tab.

NUTRITION AND DIET RESEARCH PROGRESS

IRON DEFICIENCY AND ITS COMPLICATIONS

YILDIZ DINCER
EDITOR

Nova Biomedical Books
New York

For permission to use material from this book please contact us:
Telephone 631-231-7269; Fax 631-231-8175
Web Site: http://www.novapublishers.com

Library of Congress Cataloging-in-Publication Data

Iron deficiency and its complications / editor, Yildiz Dincer.
p. ; cm.
Includes bibliographical references and index.
ISBN 978-1-61324-854-6 (hardcover)
1. Iron deficiency diseases. 2. Iron--Metabolism--Disorders. I. Dincer, Yildiz.
[DNLM: 1. Iron--deficiency. 2. Iron Metabolism Disorders--complications. 3. Iron, Dietary. WD 200.5.I7]
RC627.I75I746 2011
616.3'9--dc23

2011018628

Published by Nova Science Publishers, Inc. † New York

Contents

Preface

In the human body, iron is present in all cells and has several vital functions: as a carrier of oxygen to the tissues from the lungs in the form of hemoglobin; as a transport medium for electrons within the cells in the form of cytochromes and as an integral part of enzyme reactions in various tissues. Too little iron can interfere with these vital functions and lead to morbidity and death. This book presents current research from across the globe in the study of iron deficiency, including iron deficiency anemia in pregnant women and in gastric bypass surgery patients; the metabolic adjustment under Fe deficiency in roots of dicotyledonous plants and strategies for the fortification of food with iron.

Chapter 1 - Iron (Fe) deficiency is a yield-limiting factor for a variety of field crops grown in calcareous and alkaline soils across the world. Iron, albeit abundant, is often not soluble and therefore unavailable for root uptake. Thus, the study of processes regulating Fe uptake and translocation in plant is crucial to acquire useful knowledge to obtain biofortified plants and to improve the nutritional value of plant food that would have a dramatic positive impact on human health. Most of the plants (Strategy I) reduces soil Fe(III) to Fe(II) through a plasma membrane Fe(III)-chelate reductase, prior to takes up Fe^{2+} through a specific transporter (IRT1). However, the response to Fe deficiency stress in these plants is by far more complex than the simple activation of the reduction-based mechanism. In several Strategy I plants studied so far there is an associated increase in the activity of a plasma membrane H^+-ATPase which actively extrudes protons necessary for decreasing the rhizospheric pH and generating the electrochemical proton gradient to drive Fe uptake. Along with these activities it has been found an involvement of the metabolism to sustain the production of the reducing equivalents [NAD(P)H] and ATP. In particular, the activity of phospho*enol*pyruvate carboxylase is increased several fold. The rate of carbohydrate catabolism is also increased under these conditions and the activity of several glycolytic enzymes has been shown to be enhanced, as well. Furthermore, other metabolic pathways and free cytosolic enzymatic activities are increased during Fe deficiency, such as some cytosolic $NAD(P)^+$-dependent dehydrogenases belonging to the oxidative pentose phosphate pathway. Some of these increased activities are associated with an enhanced expression of the corresponding genes. In this chapter the authors will focus on the metabolic changes which follow the primary events involved in plant Fe uptake. The comprehension of how plants are able to adjust their metabolism under Fe starvation allows to found some inherent traits whose activation makes plants more efficient in the acquisition of this essential nutrient.

Chapter 2 - Iron deficiency (ID) remains the most prevalent single-nutrient deficiency in developing and developed countries. The World Health Organization[1] estimates that, worldwide, 1.6- 2 billion people are anemic. Although ID is responsible for at least half of the cases of anemia, there are other possible causes, including genetic, infectious, and other nutritional deficiencies. It is estimated that when anemia prevalence reaches 20%, ID exists in 50% of the population, and when anemia prevalence exceeds 40%, the entire population suffers from some degree of ID.[2] Infants, children, and women of reproductive age are at highest risk of developing ID and iron deficiency anemia (IDA), largely because of their high physiological requirements associated with growth combined with greater losses and poor dietary intake. Globally, almost half of preschool-aged children and pregnant women and close to one-third of non-pregnant women have anemia [1, 2].

Chapter 3 - Iron is a trace element, as it is required for erythropoiesis, oxidative metabolism, cellular immune response, and some of hormonal functions and enzymatic activity. Iron is distributed in the body in various compartments including hemoglobin, myoglobin, tissue iron and a labile pool. Transport of iron from one organ to another is accomplished by transferrin. The major pathway of iron metabolism is a closed cycle in which iron passes from plasma transferrin to red blood cell precursors in the bone marrow, where it is used in hemoglobin synthesis; these cells then enter the circulation in the form of mature red blood cells, where they remain nearly 120 days before they are degredated; the iron is released from hemoglobin and returns to plasma transferrin, thus completing one cycle and starting a new one. From this iron cycle, small quantities of iron are diverted for use in other iron compartments. Iron deficiency is one of the most prevalent disorder of humans. Increased iron requirements, limited external supply, and increased blood loss may lead to iron deficiency. Its causes can consist of many overlapping factor. In the initial phase of iron depletion, iron stores maintain normal levels of hemoglobin and other iron compounds. With exhaustion of iron store hypochromic and microcytic anemia becomes manifest. Iron deficiency anemia has been associated with growth retardation and lower neuronal development in infants and has long-lasting effects on mental and motor functions in spite of normalization of hematological status and growth. Adults with iron deficiency anemia have reduced attention spans and work capacity. Numerious cellular enzymes and coenzymes require iron, either as an integral part of their structure or as a cofactor. Therefore, iron is essential in various biochemical pathways required for neuronal function. Iron is required for thyroid hormon synthesis. The prevalance of iron deficiency among children living in areas of endemic goiter is high. Impaired muscle performance has been determined in iron deficiency. Chronic iron deficiency has been reported not only as a primary cause, but also as a facilitator of heart failure. Deficits in iron functional compartments have suppressive effects on the immune system. Taken together, it is clear that iron has a pivotal role in the maintenance of normal metabolic funtion and iron deficiency leads serious consequences. This chapther will review what is currently known about pathological consequences of iron deficiency and what are the mechanisms underlying these pathologies.

Chapter 4 - Anemia is a common complication in gastric surgery. It can be caused by iron, vitamin B_{12} or folate deficiency, and its prevalence may reach up to 50% of patients. Iron deficiency anemia (IDA) is the most common form of anemia and its prevalence in gastrectomized patients varies from 15 to 54%. Independently if secondary to gastrectomy used in the treatment of peptic ulcer complications and gastric cancer or to bariatric surgery for the treatment of obesity, the main causes of IDA are reduced gastric acid secretion, duodenal exclusion, inadequate intake, rapid food passage to intestine, alkaline gastritis, and Helicobacter pylori infection in the gastric remnants. Both serum iron and ferritin levels are affected by obesity and it is difficult to compare IDA prevalence in the different kinds of bariatric surgery. Patients who will be submitted or have suffered bariatric surgery deserve a careful analysis of iron status before diagnosing IDA. Although combining numerous parameters is considered the best way, serum transferrin receptor (sTfR) is very useful for the detection of IDA in the above conditions, because unlike ferritin, sTfR concentrations are not affected by the presence of inflammation. When sTfR is not available, there is some evidence that transferrin saturation rather than ferritin could be preferred to evaluate IDA in obese patients. Classically, ferrous sulfate has been used for iron deficiency anemia since the beginning of the 19th century. Since the 1980s, many studies have examined fortification of different foods with several others iron compounds, as ferrous glycynate, which is 2.5 to 3.4 fold more available than ferrous sulphate. In addition, it was hypothesized that iron amino acid chelates prevent iron from binding to inhibitors in food and, in deprived areas many developing countries, food is composed basically of rice, beans and vegetables, rich sources of phytates. Despite those hypothetical benefits, a clinical study has shown that ferrous sulphate had much more favorable results than ferrous chelate glycinate in gastrectomized patients with IDA. Parenteral iron treatment is recommended in those patients refractory to oral iron supplementation. More studies comparing different types of bariatric surgery are needed adding serum transferrin receptor or transferrin saturation as a tool to diagnose IDA prevalence.

Chapter 5 - Iron deficiency (ID) is the most common nutritional deficiency disorder in the world, affecting more than two billion people, mostly infants, children and women of childbearing age. In general, iron deficiency symptoms are attributed due to an insufficient supply of iron to the tissues, and probably not to lowered hemoglobin level. The human brain develops up until to about 20 years of age, and brain iron content also increases concomitantly up to this age. It may be difficult to repair negative effects of ID developed during this period. Several reviews and recent reports show negative effects of ID related to mental symptoms in infants and children, but unrelated to anemia; even in adolescents there exist concerns on this issue. Therefore, the outcome of current evidence strongly suggests that to assure optimal health and development, it is important to prevent and treat even mild ID of growing individuals, at least up to around 20 years of age, as well as during pregnancy. Over 200 million children worldwide do not reach their full development potential because of preventable causes, like iron deficiency. Fortification of food with iron, when an appropriate diet is not available, is considered the best sustainable way of preventing iron deficiency. The most difficult challenge to this end is to find the ideal combination of an iron fortified compound and its corresponding food vehicle. There exist many reports on the successful addition of sodium-iron ethylenediaminotetraacetate (NaFeEDTA) or ferrous bisglycinate fortifiers in the form of an iron chelate, which protects from combination with dietary inhibitors, mainly phytic acid. There is little evidence that iron fortification of staple foods, such as corn flour is a useful strategy to combat iron deficiency. However, some reports in Chile and Brazil seem to challenge this hypothesis. It could be argued that reports of marked decrease in iron absorption were verified with single meals, under special conditions, and that studies in which effects of enhancers and inhibitors of iron absorption were studied in whole meals showed results that were far less pronounced than those from single meals. Aside from these considerations, it should be emphasized that costs are very important in fortification measures, especially to convince political authorities in developing countries of the need for a continued Iron Fortification Program. Therefore, the aim of the present review is to study the different ways of fortification of food with iron in preventing and treating ID.

Chapter 6 - The aims of this research article are (i) to report new results of a population-based cohort study and (ii) to summarize the recent knowledge regarding the risk of iron deficiency anemia in pregnant women for adverse birth outcomes and the effective treatment of this pathological condition during pregnancy. The study design was the comparison the rate of preterm birth and low birthweight newborns of pregnant women with iron deficiency anemia according to the treatment of iron alone (N=1,576), iron + folic acid (N=4,419), folic acid alone (N=149) and without iron (and folic acid) treatment (N=214), in addition of pregnant women without iron deficiency anemia (N=31,793) as a reference group. Both iron deficiency anemia in pregnant women and the above adverse birth outcomes of newborns without birth defects were medically recorded in prenatal maternity logbook and discharge summary of women after delivery from inpatient obstetric clinics in the population-based Hungarian Case-Control Surveillance System of Congenital Abnormalities. There was a high rate of preterm births (15.0%) in the newborns of anemic pregnant women without iron treatment. The rate of preterm birth was only somewhat higher (10.7%) in the newborns of anemic pregnant women supplemented by iron compared to the figure of reference group (9.2%). However, anemic pregnant women with iron + folic acid treatment had a significantly lower rate of preterm births (8.2%). The secondary findings of the study are the higher prevalence of constipation, hemorrhoids and hypotension in anemic pregnant women. These findings are discussed on the basis of data in the literature. In conclusion the higher risk of preterm birth of newborn infants born to pregnant women with iron deficiency anemia can be reduced by iron treatment and prevented by iron + folic acid supplementation.

Chapter 7 - Iron deficiency is a common nutritional disorder worldwide and it is estimated that 841 000 deaths occur annually due to iron deficiency or its complication. The common causes of iron deficiency are increased demand in pregnant and growing children, poor dietary intake, and increased blood losses due to parasitic infections and disorders such as malignancy and gastrointestinal bleeding. This review article discusses the clinical and laboratory diagnosis of iron deficiency. Iron–deficient erythropoiesis will be discussed along with the key biochemical markers of iron depletion and homeostasis. The role of iron in various catalytic and selected biochemical pathways will be discussed. Storage of iron in the reticulo-endothelial system and derangements in the biochemical pathways for regulation of ferrokinetics will be discussed with emphasis on the role of membrane proteins (transferrin-transferrin receptor, hepcidin, ferroportin, etc) as well as how specific cytokines such as IL-6, TNF-α, etc, contribute to iron homeostasis. The review will also discuss the complications of iron deficiency, particularly those associated with cardiovascular, immunological and neurological disorders. The paper will discuss longitudinal studies both in humans and animal models to demonstrate neural mal-developments and long term effects of iron deficiency, including psychomotor, cognitive and affective derangements. The cardiovascular discussion of the complications of IDA will include a pathophysiological treatment of hypoxia as it affects the development of cardiomyopathy, cardiac insufficiency, hypoperfusion and angina. The risk of thrombosis associated with IDA will be discussed with particular reference to stroke occurring in children and infants. The review will also discuss the role of iron deficiency in the regulation of the immune system. In particular, the effect of iron deficiency on the production of cell-mediated and humoral immune responses and how such factors as cytokines and other products of the immune system affect the metabolism of iron will be discussed.

Chapter 8 - Short bowel syndrome, as a consequence of extended small bowel resections, lead to nutritional deficiencies. Among them, iron deserves attention. Iron replacement therapy is a challenge due to intestinal malabsorption. In this scenario, the serum iron follow-up is recommended. The objective of the present study was to assess the course of serum iron, erythrocyte and biochemical iron markers up to 960 days after extended short bowel ressections. Erythrocyte and biochemical data from 37 enterectomized patients from the15th to the 960th post-surgery day were collected, adjusted and analyzed according to a random effect model. Forty-eight percent of the patients were found to have ferritin levels below normal limits and 78% had hemoglobin concentrations below normal limits. There was a gradual increase ($p<0.05$) in serum iron after enterectomy and changes in other erythrocytes indicators ($p <0.05$). The authors conclude that although the malabsorption, short bowel syndrome patients showed increase in serum iron over time, probably due to intestinal adaptation mechanisms.

In: Iron Deficiency and Its Complications
Editor: Yildiz Dincer

ISBN 978-1-61324-854-6

Chapter 1

Metabolic Adjustment under Fe Deficiency in Roots of Dicotyledonous Plants

Gianpiero Vigani**, *Silvia Donnini and Graziano Zocchi
Dipartimento di Produzione Vegetale, Università degli Studi di Milano, Italy

Abstract

Iron (Fe) deficiency is a yield-limiting factor for a variety of field crops grown in calcareous and alkaline soils across the world. Iron, albeit abundant, is often not soluble and therefore unavailable for root uptake. Thus, the study of processes regulating Fe uptake and translocation in plant is crucial to acquire useful knowledge to obtain biofortified plants and to improve the nutritional value of plant food that would have a dramatic positive impact on human health. Most of the plants (Strategy I) reduces soil Fe(III) to Fe(II) through a plasma membrane Fe(III)-chelate reductase, prior to takes up Fe^{2+} through a specific transporter (IRT1). However, the response to Fe deficiency stress in these plants is by far more complex than the simple activation of the reduction-based mechanism. In several Strategy I plants studied so far there is an associated increase in the activity of a plasma membrane H^+-ATPase which actively extrudes protons necessary for decreasing the rhizospheric pH and generating the electrochemical proton gradient to drive Fe uptake. Along with these activities it has been found an involvement of the metabolism to sustain the production of the reducing equivalents [NAD(P)H] and ATP. In particular, the activity of phospho*enol*pyruvate carboxylase is increased several fold. The rate of carbohydrate catabolism is also increased under these conditions and the activity of several glycolytic enzymes has been shown to be enhanced, as well. Furthermore, other metabolic pathways and free cytosolic enzymatic activities are increased during Fe deficiency, such as some cytosolic $NAD(P)^+$-dependent dehydrogenases belonging to the oxidative pentose phosphate pathway. Some of these increased activities are associated with an enhanced expression of the corresponding genes. In this chapter we will focus on the metabolic changes which follow the primary events involved in plant Fe uptake. The comprehension of how plants are able to adjust

* Corresponding author: Gianpiero Vigani; E-mail: gianpiero.vigani@unimi.it

their metabolism under Fe starvation allows to found some inherent traits whose activation makes plants more efficient in the acquisition of this essential nutrient.

Keywords: ferric chelate reductase; FC-R; H^+-ATPase; organic acid; PEPC

1. INTRODUCTION

Being part of many proteins participating to fundamental mechanisms (i.e. respiration, photosynthesis and metabolism) Fe is an essential element for all the living organisms [1].

In plants most of the concern about Fe nutrition is its low availability in the soil solution due to the scarce solubility of its compounds in well aerated environment. In fact, notwithstanding its abundance, Fe exists, in well aerated soils, mainly as scarcely soluble oxides and oxi-hydroxides and therefore not freely available to plant uptake. To cope with this problem plants had developed efficient mechanisms to acquire Fe from the soil. In this context two main strategies have been developed: dicots and non-graminaceous monocots operate applying what is known as Strategy I, while graminaceous monocots operate with the Strategy II [2, 3] (Figure 1).

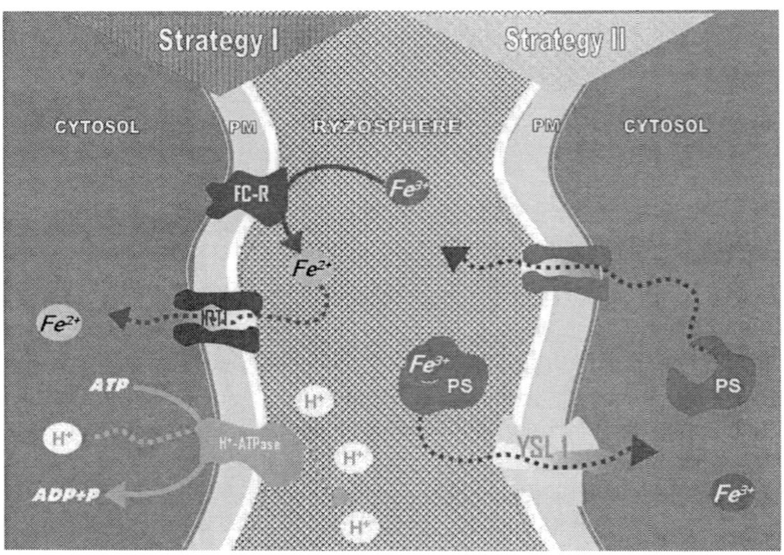

Figure 1. Schematic representation of Strategy I and Strategy II mechanisms of Fe uptake. FC-R, Ferric chelate-reductase; IRT1, Fe regulated transporter, YSL1, yellow strip like 1, PS, phytosiderophores, PM, plasmamembrane.

In Strategy I Fe acquisition is mediated by a reduction-based mechanism: a ferric chelate reductase converts Fe(III)-chelates to Fe(II) and a Fe^{2+} transporter (IRT1) moves Fe across the plasma membrane into the cell. Additionally, in most of the Strategy I plants studied so far there is an associated increase in the activity of a plasma membrane H^+-ATPase, which actively extrudes the protons necessary both for decreasing rhizospheric pH and generating the electrochemical proton gradient necessary to drive ion uptake [4,5]. The genes encoding these enzymes which characterise the Strategy I has been identified and cloned in several plants. In *Arabidopsis thaliana*, the Ferric Reductase Oxidase (*FRO2*) gene encodes the Fe deficiency inducible ferric chelate reductase that reduces Fe at the root–soil interface [6], and the *IRT1* gene encodes a high affinity Fe^{2+} transporter which transports Fe into root cells [7–8]. Putative *FRO2* and *IRT1* orthologs have been identified in a number of Strategy I species [9]. The cucumber *CsHA1* gene most probably encodes a H^{+}-ATPase that functions in Fe deficiency-induced rhizosphere acidification [10,11] (Figure 1).

By the contrast, in grasses, a group that includes most of the world's staple grain crops, a distinct strategy for Fe uptake has evolved. Grasses produce molecules of the mugineic acid family called phytosiderophores (PSs). PSs form strong hexadentate chelates with Fe(III), the predominant form of Fe found in aerobic soils. PSs are secreted into the rhizosphere where they chelate and help to solubilise Fe(III). The Fe(III)–PS complex is then taken up into root cells through the action of Yellow Stripe1 (YS1) proteins [12–13] (Figure 1).

Responses to Fe deficiency involve gene expression, a *de novo* synthesis of mRNAs and a general increase in the cellular protein content [14,15]. Several works investigating Fe deficiency responses have shown that the activities of a number of enzymes are increased which often corresponds to an increase in the protein content in addition to possible enzymatic regulation [15,16]. This has been demonstrated for IRT1, PEPC and PM-H^{+}-ATPase by western blot analysis [5,17,18,19].

Similar increases in enzymatic activities linked to organic acid metabolism [20] as well as to anaerobic [20,21] and carbohydrate [14,22,23] metabolism have also been demonstrated. Schmidt [2] showed that *de novo* synthesis of protein was required for the increased activity of the FC-R, by using the protein synthesis inhibitor cycloheximide. Furthermore, as a confirmation of this result, it has been shown that in swollen root tips, rhizodermal transfer cells have a high proportion of dense, organelle-rich cytoplasm as determined by electron microscopy analysis [15, 24, 25]. There is also clear evidence of major biosynthetic activity as the amount of polysomes extracted from Fe-deficient roots is almost double that from controls [15]. Furthermore, ^{14}C-uridine (synthesis of RNAs) and ^{14}C-leucine (protein synthesis) incorporation is higher in Fe-deficient apical roots [15]. Moreover, the amount of total amino acids was also increased in order to sustain the major protein synthesis occurring at this stage. In particular the concentrations of glutamate and aspartate were increased by 176% and 45%, respectively, as determined in cucumber roots [15]. Other biochemical activities are increased to efficiently sustain the response to Fe depletion, such as the synthesis of phenols and flavins. This chapter will focus the attention on the metabolic changes occurring on both primary and secondary matabolism which are necessary to sustain the enzymatic activities involved in Fe uptake.

2. Primary Metabolism

Fe deficiency increase the rate of NAD(P)H and ATP regeneration, since the activation of reduction processes and the enhanced proton extrusion under these conditions, require an adequate supply of energy. Several authors observed that ATP concentrations were higher under Fe deficiency [20,23] and that in bean [26] and *Plantago* roots [27] the NADH/NAD$^+$ and NADPH/NADP$^+$ redox couples became more oxidised upon addition of ferric compounds. Recharging of such substrates requires the acceleration of metabolism strictly linked to the energetic metabolism. In fact, it has been shown that the rate of glycolysis was increased [22,23] as well as the pentose phosphate pathway to both produce reducing equivalents and carbon skeleton [14,22]. In particular, the metabolic changes include: increase in the activity of PEPC and of several enzymes of the glycolytic pathway such as glyceraldehyde 3-phosphate dehydrogenase (GAPDH), pyruvate kinase (PK) and ATP-dependent phosphofructokinase (ATP-PFK1) and of the Krebs cycle such as citrate synthase, isocitrate dehydrogenase, fumarase and aconitase [20,28]. Some of these increased activities are associated with an enhanced expression of the corresponding genes [29]. Several studies reports findings supporting these data both at proteomic and biochemical level [28 and reference therein].

The mains processes responsible to adjust the changing energy demand under stress condition are glycolysis and mitochondrial pathways.

2.1. Glycolysis

In plant roots glucose is the primary source for carbon skeleton supply and for the energetic substrates synthesis. In the roots, the elevated requirement of glucose is maintained by translocation of photosynthate from the shoot or by degrading starch stores. In fact, in bean plants [30] the sugar concentration was doubled with respect to the control in the phloem sap of Fe-deficient plants. Accordingly, microarray analysis showed that in *Arabidopsis* shoots the genes encoding α-amylase synthesis, the Pi translocator and the H$^+$-sucrose symporter were induced after three days of Fe starvation [29]. In Fe-deficient cucumber roots, the carbohydrate concentration (particularly glucose 6-phosphate and fructose 6-phosphate) has been reported to increase while the quantity of starch was greatly decreased [23]. Futhermore, under these conditions, several glycolytic enzymes, such as hexokinase (HK), ATP-PFK 1, GAPDH and PK activities [22, 23, 31], have been shown to be activated increasing the rate of carbohydrate catabolism [14, 22, 23]. These responses are likely associated with enhanced gene expression [29]. Recently, several proteomic studies have been performed on Strategy I plants [32,33]. In cucumber roots twenty-one proteins are over accumulated under Fe deficiency. Among these, the majority (42%) are enzymes belonging to the glycolytic pathway (e.g. PP-dependent phosphofructokinase (PP-PFK), aldolase, phosphoglycerate kinase (PGK), phosphoglycerate mutase (PGM) and enolase) confirming previous biochemical data suggesting the involvement of metabolism, and in particular of glycolysis, in response to Fe deficiency [32]. Also, Rellan-Alvarez et al., [33] in *Beta vulgaris* roots reported further data supporting the activation of glycolysis under Fe deficiency at the protein level and at the metabolic level, as well. Most of the proteins found to be over-accumulated in sugar beet tips under Fe deficiency were identified as enzymes of the carbohydrate catabolism, including 5 out of the 10 glycolytic enzymes (fructose 1,6-bisphosphate aldolase, triosephosphate isomerase, glyceraldehyde 3-phosphate dehydrogenase, 3-phosphoglycerate kinase and enolase), one of the citric acid cycle, malate dehydrogenase (MDH) and fructokinase. Increase in the activities and concentration of several glycolytic enzymes in root extract of Fe-deficient plants have been previously found, including fructose 1,6-bisphosphate aldolase, enolase, triosephosphate isomerase and GADPH [33 and references therein].

In Fe-deficient tomato root, the expression of four enzymes (UDP-glucose pyrophosphorylase precursor, UDP-glucose dehydrogenase 2, trehalose-phosphatase, and cytosolic phosphoglucomutase), which are involved in the starch degradation, were increased [34]. Additionally, glucan endo-1,3-β-D-glucosidase and sucrose synthase, which catalyze reactions more closely with sucrose and glucan synthesis, were also decreased. These data obviously supported that the starch degradation process was enhanced and the sucrose and glucan metabolism was down-regulated in tomato roots under Fe deficiency [34].

Up-regulation of glycolysis provides: i) ATP synthesis to sustain the major activity of the H^+-ATPase; ii) formation of reducing equivalents for the FC-R; iii) formation of phospho*enol*pyruvate (PEP), iv) a contribution to the regulation of cytosolic pH (see below). Furthermore, other metabolic pathways and free cytosolic enzymatic activities are up-regulated during Fe deficiency. In particular, some cytosolic $NAD(P)^+$-dependent dehydrogenases such as glucose 6-phosphate dehydrogenase (oxidative pentose phosphate pathway) [14,20,22], malic enzyme [14,22], glyceraldehyde 3-phosphate dehydrogenase [14,22,23], and isocitrate dehydrogenase [20] showed increased activity in order to produce reducing equivalents necessary to keep the FC-R working at the operative rate. Microarray data presented by Thimm *et al.* (2001) partially agree with the conclusions from biochemical analyses. However, in *Arabidopsis*, microarray studies revealed changes in expression levels of only a few of the above-mentioned enzymes during Fe deficiency. This does not necessarily contrast with the biochemical data obtained in other plant species; in fact, cucumber roots, for example, behave for some responses quite differently from *Arabidopsis* used in that study and many responses to environmental changes are likely to be mediated at the post-translational level and thus not detectable at the level of transcription. The importance of rhizosphere acidification in the responses of Strategy I plants to Fe deficiency has been recognised for many years [35]. This response has been associated with the activity of a plasma membrane localised H^+-ATPase [35]. However, unlike the FC-R, increased H^+-ATPase activity was not always observed and the extent of stimulation of the enzyme activity seemed to differ considerably among plant species and genotypes, ranging from a very low value to about 100% [2]. In cucumber roots, one of the most active acidifying species, it has been shown by blotting analysis that the development of a higher activity under Fe deficiency was associated with an increase in the level of the enzyme [5] and of its transcript [37].

Among the metabolic activities that are increased under Fe deficiency, phosphor-*enol*pyruvate carboxylase (PEPC) is considered one of the most important. PEPC is an ubiquitous enzyme in plants which catalyses the fixation of bicarbonate to phospho*enol*pyruvate to produce oxaloacetate and Pi. In non-photosynthetic tissues PEPC acts in several anaplerotic reactions: i) to replenish tricarboxylic acid cycle intermediates, ii) to provide carbon skeletons to sustain the synthesis of amino acids during NH_4^+ assimilation and iii) for the regulation of cytoplasmic pH. In Fe-deficient cucumber roots [17] and in the yellow zone of Fe-deficient sugar beet roots [20] PEPC activity was, respectively, four and sixty times higher than in control roots. The PEPC increased activity is attributable to increases in protein expression [17] and by induction of mRNA transcription [37]. The significance of PEPC activity increase might be explained by two hypotheses. The first one follows the pH-stat theory formulated by Davies [38], in which cytoplasm alkalinisation associated with proton extrusion would in turn activate PEPC activity to produce organic acids. This activation was interpreted as a major effort of the biochemical pH-stat system to re-equilibrate the cytosolic pH to its physiological value. This speculation was in part confirmed by an *in vivo* ^{31}P-NMR study which showed that the pH_c was effectively increased under Fe deficiency [23]. The second hypothesis suggests a more complex role for PEPC. Increased glycolysis observed in Fe-deficient root seems to be the pathway responsible to satisfy both ATP and H^+ production to keep the H^+-ATPase working. To maintain the rate of glycolysis sufficiently high, PEP must be consumed at a high rate, as well. Its utilisation can be carried out by PK and/or by PEPC. Consumption of PEP relieves its own allosteric inhibition on the key glycolytic enzyme PFK 1. Furthermore, the PEPC activity increases Pi concentration thus activating PFK 1 by relieving the inhibition by PEP [28]. In plants where the H^+-ATPase activity is high (for instance, cucumber roots), the activity of the PEPC has been shown to be very high, and as a consequence the rate of glycolysis is increased. Generally, the PEPC activation could be the driving downstream force for glycolysis leading to an its increase in the rate and producing cytosolic acidification that would in turn activate the H^+-ATPase. Moreover, the activation of PEPC could be responsible for the production of organic acids. It has been shown that under Fe deficiency, plants often produce substantial amounts of organic acids, particularly citrate and malate [39 and references therein]. Two important roles might be attributed to these organic acids. The former will carry out chelation and transport of Fe within the plant (vascular transport). The latter involves several aspects of metabolism.

Interestingly, since the production of organic acids is protogenic, it might thus be useful in controlling the cytosolic pH or to feed the increased activity of the PM H^+-ATPase. Furthermore, elevated production of oxaloacetate and/or malate could be used to replenish the Krebs cycle. This anaplerotic function is important to keep the cycle working with a limiting concentrations of pyruvate to produce both ATP and citrate. These can be exported from mitochondria to accomplish both the chemical and biochemical cytosolic functions. In fact, they can be extruded from the roots to facilitate acquisition of Fe from the soil or transported to the shoot via the xylem. Interestingly, citrate could provide carbon skeletons to chlorotic leaves to sustain growth and respiration [39]. On the other hand, citrate could be used to produce reducing equivalents for the FC-R through the action of the cytosolic $NADP^+$-dependent isocitrate dehydrogenase (ICDH) and production of 2-oxoglutarate [28]. Since it has been shown that protein synthesis is increased (see below) under Fe deficiency and that this requires synthesis of amino acids, 2-oxoglutarate and the same product of PEPC, oxaloacetate, could be used in nitrogen assimilation thus linking the metabolism of carbon with that of nitrogen.

2.2. Mitochondria

Aerobic respiration is a process common to almost all eukaryotic organism releasing a large amount of free energy and it is confined to the mitochondria. Mitochondria possess two membranes that divide the organelle into four compartments: the outer membrane, the region between the two membranes (intermembrane space), a highly invaginated inner membrane, and the aqueous phase, the matrix, contained within the inner membrane. The enzymatic complexes belonging to respiratory chain are localised within the inner membrane, whereas the tricarboxylic acid cycle (TCA or Krebs cycle) takes place in the matrix [40]. Both the mitochondrial respiration and TCA are essential processes for the cell life. Fe deficiency and mitochondria are topic strongly linked each other, mainly for two reasons. Firstly, as stated before, Fe deficiency greatly induce the Strategy I activities leading to a strong energy request. Secondly, mitochondria could be consider a Fe-dependent compartment of the cell. In fact, several enzymes belonging both to the respiratory chain and to the Krebs cycle are Fe-containing proteins (Figure 2). Moreover, crucial steps in the Fe-S cluster assembly of the whole cell takes place in mitochondria, suggesting the important role of this compartment in Fe handling of the cell.

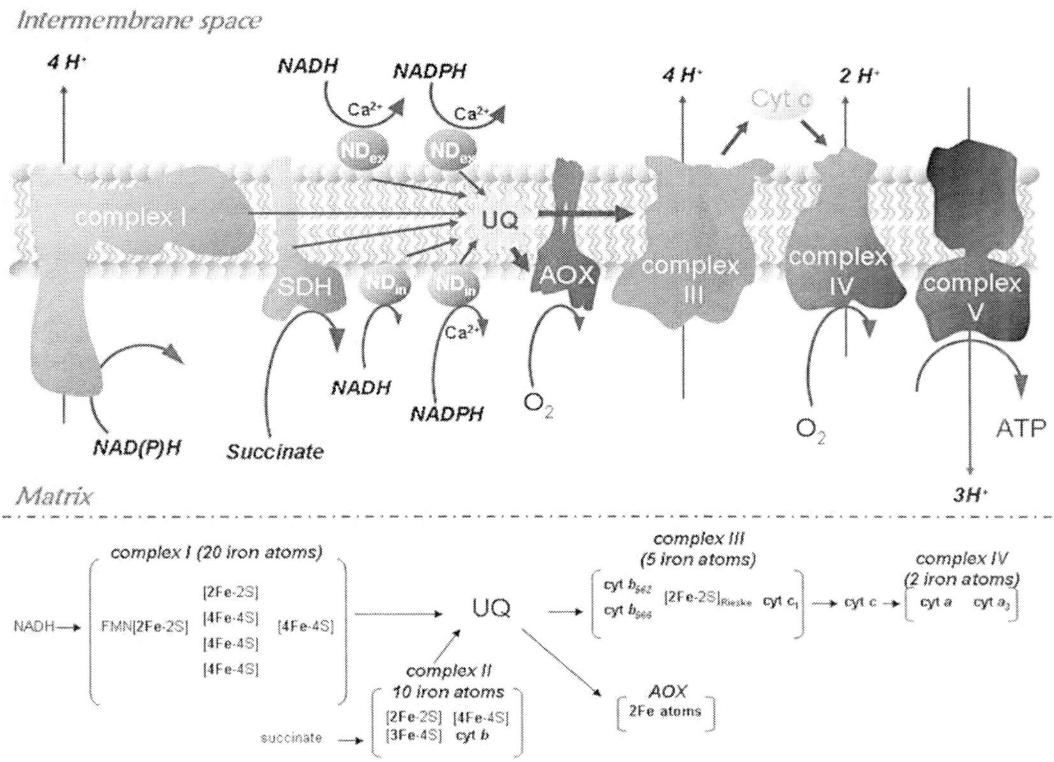

Figure 2. Representation of Fe distribution and Fe content in the complexes of plant respiratory chain. Complex I contains 20 Fe atoms, Complex II contains 10 Fe atoms, Complex III contains 5 Fe atoms, Complex IV contains 2 Fe atoms and AOX contains 2 Fe atoms. AOX, alternative oxidase ; UQ, ubiquinone pool.

In this section the effects of Fe deficiency on both respiratory chain and TCA activities in roots will be discussed.

In mitochondria of all eukaryotes, the principal respiratory electron transfer chain consist of a series of membrane-bound redox centres that catalyze the multi-step transfer of electrons from NADH and $FADH_2$ to oxygen, forming water and releasing energy, which is used to translocate protons from the matrix to the intermembrane spaces. The electron transfer chain facilitates a number of modestly exergonic redox reactions, rather than a single explosive one, and conserves energy through proton translocation. The F_1F_0 ATP synthase provides a path for passive proton diffusion into the matrix and uses the free energy released by this spontaneous diffusion to drive the phosphorylation of ADP. In addition to the electron transfer chain shared by all aerobic eukaryotes, plant mitochondria also possess novel pathways for both the oxidation of NADH and the reduction of oxygen. These unique bypass proteins, the so called alternative NAD(P)H dehydrogenases and the alternative oxidase (AOX) do not pump protons and the free energy released by the electron flow through them is lost as heat. The standard mitochondrial electron transfer chain consist of four multi-centered protein complexes, commonly referred to as Complex I through IV. The F_1F_0-ATP synthase, which does not have electron transfer activity, is referred to as Complex V. Complex I is an NADH dehydrogenase that oxidizes the NADH generated in the mitochondrial matrix by the TCA cycle, regenerating NAD^+ and reducing ubiquinone. Complex II, which contains a component enzyme of the citric acid cycle (succinate dehydrogenase), oxidizes succinate to fumarate. Like Complex I, Complex II transfers electrons to ubiquinone. Ubiquinone can carry one or two electrons. Both fully oxidized ubiquinone and ubiquinol molecules are highly hydrophobic and capable of transverse and lateral movements within the inner membrane [40 and references therein].

At respiratory chain level, the enzymatic complexes of the mitochondrial electron transport chain (mtETC) contain several Fe-S cluster and heme groups [28,41]. In the absence of Fe, heme and Fe-S cluster synthesis should be impaired and indeed the *de novo* synthesis of Fe-containing proteins occurs at a lower rate in mitochondria of Fe deficient plants [28]. In fact, it has been shown that the level of some Fe containing components (cytochromes and Fe-S clusters) were greatly diminished in mitochondria of Fe-deficient sycamore cells [42] and cucumber roots [41].

Moreover, in cucumber root it has been shown that the number of Fe ions required for the correct assembly of each mtETC complexes and their relative activities in Fe-deficient conditions are strongly correlated: complex IV, which has only two Fe, shows a decrease by about 50%; while complex I and II, which require, at least, 20 and 10 Fe atoms, respectively, show a stronger decrease (95% and 77%, respectively). Taken together, these data suggest that in Fe-limiting condition, mitochondria could preferentially allocate Fe to complexes III and IV rather than to complexes I and II. Thus Fe-deficient mitochondria seem to become the biggest 'victim' of the Fe starvation in root tissues, requiring at least 40 Fe atoms/respiratory unit to work [41]. As stated before, plant mitochondria are characterized by the presence of several alternative pathways which are able to oxidise reducing equivalents, such as alternative NAD(P)H dehydrogenases (ND-DHs) [43,44]. Distinct external rotenone-insensitive enzymes oxidise cytoplasmic NADH and NADPH in a calcium-dependent manner (ND_{ex}) [45]. Matrix NADH can be oxidised via two alternative enzymes. NADH oxidation through the rotenone-sensitive complex I mediates ATP production via proton pumping, whereas the activity of the rotenone-insensitive NADH dehydrogenases (ND_{in}) is not restricted by coupling to energy conservation [46]. Additionally, a calcium-dependent rotenone-insensitive NADPH dehydrogenase is present at the matrix surface of the inner membrane [47,48]. In cucumber roots it has been observed that in Fe-deficient mitochondria the ND_{ex} are strongly induced with respect to the ND_{in}, concerning both the enzymatic activity and the protein level [49]. These findings suggest that, through the ND_{ex}, the respiratory chain can contribute to the cytosolic NAD(P)H turnover, notwithstanding the mtETC is strongly affected by Fe deficiency. The increase of ND_{in} activities, in Fe-deficient mitochondria, is not supported by the induction of the relative protein content, suggesting the presence of a post-translational regulation. The lower induction of the ND_{in} activities with respect to the ND_{ex} could be related to a lower request of NAD(P)H turnover from the matrix than from the cytosol.

However, a proteomic investigation performed on Fe-deficient *Arabidopsis* roots showed that several protein belonging to respiratory chain accumulated more than in control condition [50] such as, the cytochrome c oxidase, the ubiquinol-cytochrome c reductase complex ubiquinone-binding protein and three component of mitochondrial complex I. The contrasting results obtained in cucumber respect to *Arabidopsis* plant might be explained by the different degree of Fe deficiency condition used.

At the level of the mitochondrial matrix the knowledge about Krebs cycle reported in the literature suggests that Fe deficiency induces an activation of the process. In *Beta vulgaris* a metabolomic study revealed large increases in organic acids, including a 20-fold citric acid increase [33]. These increases in the organic acids of TCA cycle under Fe deficiency are coupled with increases in glycolysis [20,34] and root CO_2 fixation by PEPC [17,51], and provide an anaplerotic, non-autotrophic (via xylem) C source for leaves which have otherwise reduced the photosynthetic rates [52,53].

Li and coworkers [34] observed several enzymes (isocitrate dehydrogenase (NADP1), aconitase, succinyl CoA ligase, succinate dehydrogenase) belonging to the TCA cycle which revealed simultaneously up-regulated expression under Fe deficiency in tomato roots. Furthermore, ATP- citrate lyase, which lowers TCA cycle, was decreased. Meanwhile, PEPC, a key enzyme catalyzing phospho*enol*pyruvate to form oxaloacetate as carbon source for TCA cycle, was increased. The results strongly supported that the mitochondrial TCA cycle was enhanced in response to Fe deficiency. In López-Millán et al., [54] total organic anion concentrations in tomato root tips did not change significantly with Fe deficiency, but the composition of the organic anion pool was markedly changed. In control root tips, the major organic anions (more than 90% of the total organic anion concentration) were oxalate, 2-oxoglutarate and malate, whereas in Fe-deficient root tips citrate and malate accounted for 90% of the total organic anion concentration. Moreover, the authors observed that Fe deficiency led to a major (20-fold) increase in citrate concentration and to large decrease in the concentrations of 2-oxoglutarate, oxalate and malate (96%, 90% and 67%, respectively). Low concentrations of cis-aconitate and fumarate were also detected in tomato root tips, but concentrations did not change significantly as a result of Fe shortage. The authors also measured five enzymatic activities involved in organic acid metabolism in tissue extracts. All of them increased significantly in the extract of Fe-deficient root tips when compared with that obtained from Fe-sufficient ones. Increases were 10.5-fold for ICDH, 7.2-fold for aconitase, 4.9-fold for MDH, 3.5-fold for fumarase and 2.3-fold for citrate synthase (CS). Changes found in the organic acid pool in tomato roots under Fe deficiency are likely associated with the increase in PEPC activity, which is accompanied by increases in the activities of several enzymes involved in organic acid synthesis, including MDH, CS, ICDH, aconitase and fumarase (4.9-, 2.3-, 10.5-, 7- and 3.5-fold, respectively). PEPC catalyses the carboxylation of PEP to oxalacetate, which could subsequently be reduced to malate via cytosolic MDH. Malate could then be transported to mitochondria via malate–oxalacetate shuttle and enter the Krebs cycle [54]. The authors pointed out that the up-regulation of TCA cycle might have special significance for roots in response to Fe deficiency. TCA cycle provides abundant organic acids including citrate and malate which play an important role as chelators for Fe transport in plants [52, 55]. Furthermore, also proteomic data indicated that the TCA cycle was enhanced under Fe deficiency and these are in agreement with the transcriptional data in *Arabidopsis* [29], the increased enzyme activity involved in organic acid metabolism in sugar beet [20], and the increased organic acids in xylem sap of sugar beet upon Fe deficiency [52]. TCA is the biochemical and physiological basis for increased extrusion of organic acids in Fe-deficient root. Acidification of the rhizosphere upon Fe limitation needs proton secretion. The organic acids produced by TCA cycle should also be the source for it. All the data suggest that TCA cycle plays important roles in Fe deficiency response to provide organic acids and protons.

All the papers published reporting an enhancement of TCA under Fe deficiency showed, actually, results obtained on total protein extract and not on purified mitochondria loosing the discrimination between the same reactions occurring both in mitochondrial matrix and cytosol (i.e. reactions catalysed by aconitase, ICDH, MDH). Like the respiratory chain, also the TCA posses two Fe-containing enzymes (i.e. the aconitase and the succinate dehydrogenase (Complex II of respiratory chain)). Interestingly, Complex II or succinate dehydrogenase activity determined in purified mitochondria obtained from cucumber roots [41] and from sycamore cells [42] strongly decreased under Fe deficiency, suggesting that, at least in a single point, the TCA decelerate.

Said that, these data suggest the complexity of the metabolic responses to Fe deficiency occurring at TCA level and more work must be done to clearly define the real metabolic regulation .

Fe deficiency affects also the morphology and the ultrastructure of the mitochondria. In fact, mitochondria from Fe-deficient sycamore cells displayed a more dilute matrix with less pronounced cristae consistent with the marked decline in cytochromes and Fe-S clusters [42]. Interestingly, in Fe-deficient cucumber roots, mitochondria displayed a particular handlebar-like structure and they seem to aggregate each others [41].

The higher plant chondriome (all the mitochondria in a cell, collectively) is a highly dynamic structure composed predominantly by physically discrete organelles. This structure contrasts with that of most animal cell types and yeast cells where the chondriome is frequently organised into long tubules or reticula. Analysis of mitochondrial morphology *in vivo* has shown that higher plant mitochondria are highly pleomorphic, although most frequently they are spherical to sausage-shaped organelles. In general, the morphology of mitochondria is very dynamic, often changing shape within a cell and from one cell type to another. Mitochondria are also dynamic, in terms of their movement within cells, moving rapidly along cellular structures, such as actin and microtubule cytoskeleton [59]. The main mitochondrial processes that regulate the shape and the movement of the organelles in the cell are the fusion and the fission. These two processes compensate each other leading to the maintenance of a relatively constant number of mitochondria in the cells [59]. When mitochondrial fusion predominates, mitochondria become highly interconnected or networked. On the contrary, fragmentation of mitochondria and inhibition of fusion accompany the earliest steps of mitochondria-mediated apoptosis. Several authors suggest that the number of mitochondria are enhanced in Fe-deficient cells [24,42,56,57] so we might hypothesize that this nutritional stress could bring to a modification of the mitochondrial fusion/fission ratio. Moreover, a similar handlebar-like structure observed in Fe-deficient cucumber root has been also observed in *Arabidopsis* DRP3A mutant [59]. Until now there is not specific evidence about a possible impairment of fusion and fission processes under Fe deficiency, but the change in the number [29], in the shape [41] and in the ultrastructure [42] of mitochondria suggests that a low availability of Fe, by altering *de novo* synthesis of Fe-S clusters and heme containing proteins, impairs the mitochondrial dynamic processes.

2.3. Reprogramming of Primary Metabolism

Since the maintenance of FC-R and H^+-ATPase activities requires the constant production of energetic substrates, also the metabolism has been studied under Fe deficiency condition. Furthermore, the PEPC activity sustains the anaplerotic production of carbon skeleton for biosynthetic pathways (in particular the synthesis of amino acids) and along with the accumulation of di-tricarboxylic acid carrier (DTC) increases the communication between the cytosolic and the mitochondrial pool of organic acids to help to maintain a higher turnover of reducing equivalents [41]. Implication of metabolism has been also inferred from the microarray analysis performed on Fe-starved *Arabidopsis* plants [29], in which it was shown that the level of several transcripts encoding enzymes of these metabolic pathways were increased. Organic acids are important for the translocation of Fe throughout the plant, as source of carbon skeleton and for the regulation of cytosolic pH [20,54]. The increased organic acid flux between cytosol and mitochondria could be a strategy of the cell to allow a faster turnover of reducing equivalents [41,60]. Since both the cytosolic and the mitochondrial NAD(P)H need to be re-oxidized to keep the catabolic pathways working, a less efficient respiratory chain activity could impair this turnover, leading to a higher ratio of reduced over oxidized pyridine nucleotides, as showed in bean for NADPH/$NADP^+$ ratio [26]. A lower turnover rate might in turn decrease the rate of other metabolic pathways (for instance glycolysis) causing an imbalance of energy and metabolite production. However, in *Plantago lanceolata* the total pool of pyridine nucleotides was more oxidized under Fe deficiency, although the NADPH/$NADP^+$ pool was slightly higher [27]. On the contrary, the NAD(P)H/$NAD(P)^+$ ratio was lower in Fe-deficient sugar beet and tomato roots with respect to the control [20,54]. Taken together, these data show how complex is the balance between the reducing and oxidising processes and that Fe deficiency strongly induces the NAD(P)H oxidising activities over the $NAD(P)^+$ reducing activities.

The great production of reduced NAD(P)H from the metabolism need to be oxidised allowing its turnover in cell. Considering that the respiratory chain is affected by Fe deficiency, the reactions of the cell capable to consume NAD(P)H are the FC-R and the anaerobic pathway. Indeed López-Millán et al., [20,54] reported that Fe deficiency increased the fermentative enzyme activities such as lactate dehydrogenase (LDH) and pyruvate decarboxylase (PDC) and several other cytosolic NADH-consuming enzymes, that could contribute to the oxidation of the pyridine nucleotide pool in tomato and sugar beet roots. These data are also confirmed by microarray analysis on Fe-deficient *Arabidopsis* [29] and by proteomic data obtained from cucumber root, in which putative alcohol dehydrogenase and malate dehydrogenase proteins accumulated under Fe deficiency [32]. However it is important to not exclude the mitochondria from being able to carry out any oxidative process of reduced pyridine nucleotides. Indeed, also the mitochondria might participate in the oxidation of NAD(P)H under Fe deficiency by the activation of their alternative pathways: NAD(P)H DHs activities seem to be activated to bypass the strong loss of Complex I and Complex II activities occurring in Fe-deficient cucumber roots. The external and internal localization of these enzymes in the inner mitochondrial membrane allow them to oxidize the

NAD(P)H from both the cytosol and the matrix side, but until now, however, there is no evidence supporting their involvement under Fe deficiency. Concerning the AOX activity, in the literature there are only indirect data relative to the oxygraph analysis in which the SHAM-sensitive pathway decrease in Fe-deficient root tissues with respect to the control. [20, 41,54].

Moreover, the cytosolic reducing equivalents may be transferred to mitochondria through several metabolite shuttles that operate between the two compartments (i.e malate/ oxaloacetate [61], malate/aspartate [62], and the glycerol-3-phosphate (G-3-P) [63,64].

Fe deficiency induces, from one hand, a great enhancement of FC-R and H^+-ATPase activities, leading to a strong request of energy in the form of NAD(P)H and ATP and from the other hand a limitation of mitochondrial functionality, lowering the efficiency of the main cellular site of energy production.

Thus, Fe deficiency leads to the coexistence of two contrasting metabolic aspects: a strong energy demand versus a strong limitation of mitochondria activity, establishing a kind of energetic emergency status of the cell. To survive under Fe-limiting growing condition the cell must find alternative energy producing mechanisms. In this contest, glycolysis could represent a first aid for the cell to avoid the cellular energetic collapse. As postulated in Vigani et al., (2009) Fe deficiency could simulate a kind of "cellular effort" in which to overcome a respiratory chain impairment, the cell needs alternative pathways to sustain both energetic requirements and NAD(P)H turnover. The cell could then enable *a*) glycolytic and anaerobic pathways to run faster, to sustain ATP synthesis, and, *b*) organic acid exchange between mitochondria and cytosol to sustain NAD(P)H turnover and carbon flux [41] (Figure 3).

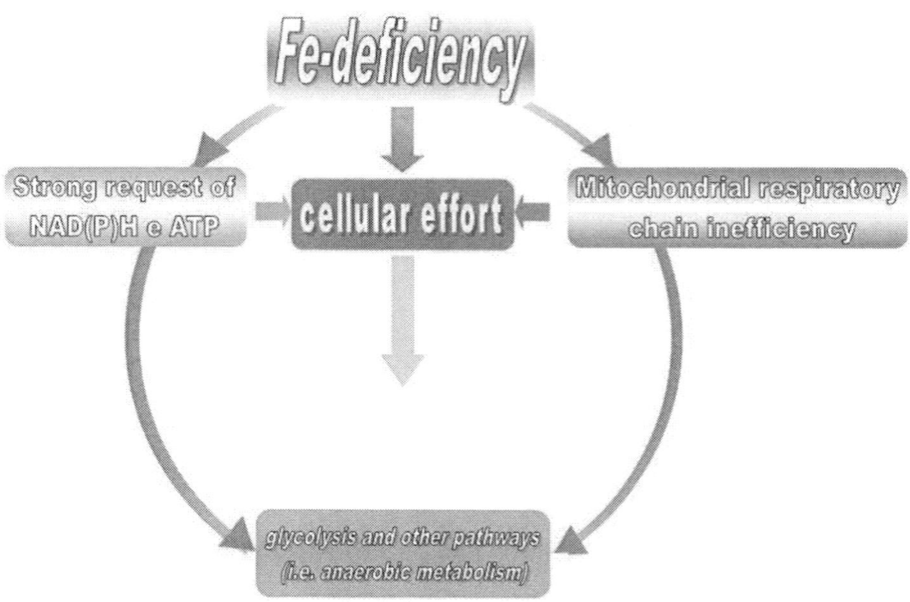

Figure 3. Schematic representation of the primary metabolism reprogramming of Fe-deficient plant roots. Fe deficiency induces both a strong energetic request and a mitochondrial inefficiency. The coexistence of these two contrasting metabolic aspects simulate a kind of "cellular effort". To overcome this condition, cell activate glycolysis and other pathways (i.e. anaerobic metabolism).

3. Secondary Metabolism

Some Strategy I species are able to release organic compounds like phenols, flavins and organic acids in the soil helpful in the solubilisation of Fe containing compounds [3, 54, 65, 66]. However, their mechanism of action and their importance in the Fe acquisition is not yet completely understood.

Phenols compared with other compounds in root exudates, are particularly interesting because of their multiple functions, such as Fe chelation, reduction and radical scavenging.

M'Sehli et al. [67] showed in *Medicago ciliaris* an accumulation of phenols under Fe deficiency, in agreement with previous results obtained in tomato [68] and in *Parietaria diffusa* [69]. Concerning *M. ciliaris*, the concentration of phenols in Fe-deficient tissues underwent a significant increase, especially when Fe deficiency was induced by bicarbonate. Moreover, a higher content was found in the tolerant line (TN11.11) than in the sensible one (TN8.7). The presence of high concentration of bicarbonate in the hydroponic culture induced a strong increase in phenols also in *Parietaria* roots [69]. In this case, a moderate increase was found in the presence of low concentration of bicarbonate, while in plants grown in the absence of Fe the increase in sugar concentration was accompanied by a decrease in phenol content. *Parietaria* plants grown in the presence of bicarbonate showed the formation of proteoid-like roots. These structures, developing from secondary and tertiary lateral roots provide an enhanced surface of contact between plant and soil useful for the release of nutrient-solubilising compounds (e.g. phenols) and for the acquisition of the nutrients from the rhizosphere [70]. In *Parietaria* the presence of such structures only in plants grown with bicarbonate supply suggested that this should not be a specific response to Fe deficiency but, more likely, to a more general condition of low nutrient availability (for instance P) typical of this growth condition.

Despite the fact the phenols are usually reported to be the main components of root exudates, relatively little is known about their role in Fe nutrition. It has been suggested that the released phenolic compounds function to enhance Fe availability in the rhizosphere as an alternative/supplement to the plasma membrane-bound ferric chelate reductase, FC-R [71]. Recent literature [72], demonstrated that phenolic compounds can play a critical role in facilitating the reutilization of apoplastic Fe in roots. The cell wall, the major component of root apoplast, contains highly negatively charged sites that can serve as a sink for most cationic mineral nutrients. Under Fe deficiency Fe desorption from the cell wall could be achieved by the chemical means of chelation and reduction performed by the phenols themselves. This was supported by the observation that removal of phenols significantly enhanced root FC-R activity, which is normally induced by plant Fe deficiency.

Phenolic compounds can be increased or *de novo* synthesized not only under Fe deficiency condition, but also as a response to other nutrient deficiencies. In these stress conditions, plants growth is reduced compared to control while net photosynthesis is not as sensitive. Thus, carbohydrates accumulated could be diverted into secondary metabolism [73] to produce phenols [74]. Both the oxidative pentose phosphate pathway and Calvin cycle can provide carbon skeletons in form of erythrose-4-phosphate, which together with phospho*enol*pyruvate formed from glycolysis can be used as precursors for phenylpropanoid metabolism via the shikimic acid pathway (Figure 4).

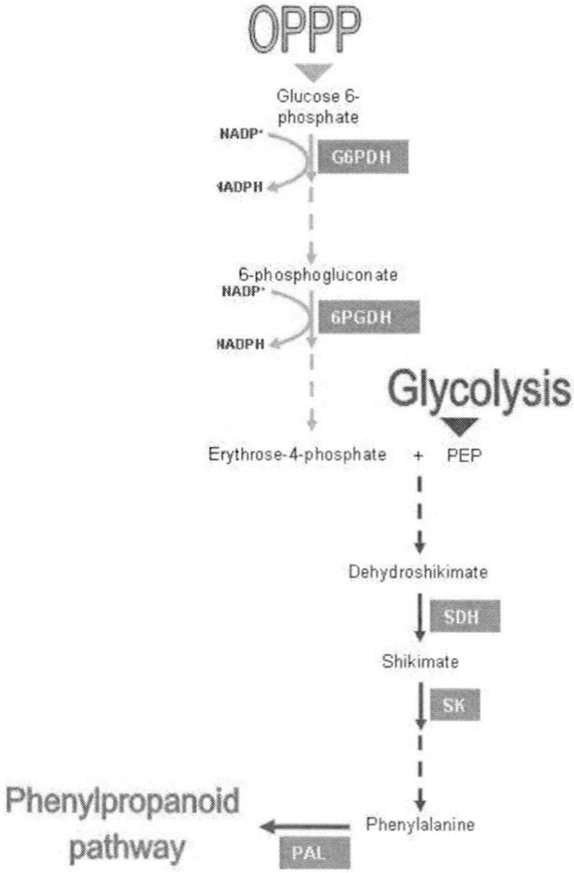

Figure 4. Scheme showing the relationships between primary and secondary metabolism. The phenylpropanoid metabolism *via* the shikimic acid pathway is shown. OPPP: oxidative pentose phosphate pathway; G6PDH: Glucose-6-phosphate dehydrogenase (EC 1.1.1.49); 6PGDH: 6-Phosphogluconate dehydrogenase (EC 1.1.1.44); SDH: Shikimate dehydrogenase (EC 1.1.1.25); SK: Shikimate Kinase (EC 2.7.1.71); PAL: Phenylalanine ammonia-lyase (EC 4.3.1.5).

The observed stimulatory effect of Fe deficiency on the total phenol content led to investigate on the activity of three enzymes belonging to the shikimate pathway involved in phenols synthesis: shikimate kinase (SK), shikimate dehydrogenase (SDH) and phenylalanine ammonia lyase (PAL).

The shikimate pathway converts simple carbohydrates to aromatic amino acids, such as phenylalanine, which is the first substrate for the phenylpropanoid pathway. Phenylalanine is required for the synthesis of various phenolic compounds [75]. PAL (a key enzyme in phenylpropanoid pathway) is widely distributed in plants and is believed to be the main enzyme responsible for phenols synthesis, conferring increased tolerance to a wide array of stresses [76]. The activation of phenylpropanoid pathway by biotic stress is well established [77, 78]. However, the ability of a wide range of abiotic stresses to stimulate phenylpropanoid pathway is less appreciated. These include high light [79], low temperature [80], phosphate deficiency [81] and aluminium toxicity [82].

Studies on *Medicago ciliaris* [67] grown under Fe deficiency showed an increase in the PAL activity and in the activity of some of the key enzymes catalyzing the biosynthesis of phenols such as SDH and SK. Moreover, the work demonstrates that the different Fe deficiency tolerance found in two *Medicago* lines (tolerant TN11.11 and sensible TN8.7) can be ascribed to the different aptitude to increase secondary metabolism pathways, leading to more efficient Fe mobilization and reducing oxidative damage. In agreement, the results obtained in *Parietaria* (Donnini et al., unpublished) showed that there was a good correlation between the increase in phenol compounds in the roots and the increase in the phenol biosynthesis pathway; in fact, the enhanced activity of the SDH and PAL, as well as the enhanced amount of phenolic compounds were found in both Fe-deficient conditions, but more under the bicarbonate treatment.

In non-graminaceous monocots and dicots, phenolic compounds are frequently reported to be the main components of root exudates in response to Fe deficiency. Additionally, organic acid and/or riboflavin secretion induced by Fe deficiency has also been occasionally reported [83, 84]. Fe-deficient plants accumulate organic acids in roots, xylem sap, leaf apoplastic fluid and whole leaves [85, 20]. Moreover, the excretion of organic acids from roots into the rhizosphere was reported under Fe deficiency [86, 87]. The role of organic acid is essential in making the scarcely soluble soil Fe available to growing plants [88, 89, 90]. Citrate and malate are the main carboxylate anions accumulating in the root tissues and exudates in response to Fe deficiency [91, 92, 93].

M'sehli et al. [67] showed that the total pool of organic anions (citrate and malate) was higher in Fe-deficient *Medicago* roots with respect to the control. However, the highest value of organic acid concentration was found in the tolerant genotype, characterized also by a high proton extrusion activity, as reported before for grapevine [93], woody species [91, 92] and herbaceous plants [39]. Since citrate accumulation is generally more pronounced than malate, citrate could be taken into consideration as a biochemical marker of Fe chlorosis tolerance, as suggested by Ollat et al. [93] and Rombolà et al. [92] for other species. Lambers et al. [94] and Veneklaas et al. [95] found that the proportion of malate to citrate in the rhizosphere varied as a function of soil pH.

In *Parietaria* roots (Donnini et al., unpublished) both malic and citric acid content, expressed on a fresh weight basis, was found to increase as Fe in the hydroponic culture was removed. However, when bicarbonate was added to the control solution, the amount of organic acid in the roots was significantly higher. Interestingly, the malic acid content in the exudates of plants grown in the absence of Fe was significantly higher than plants grown with bicarbonate supply, while was the contrary for citric acid, being the content strongly increased in the presence of bicarbonate. The increased organic acid pools in Fe-deficient roots could be linked to a coordinated increase in the activities of PEPC and MDH. PEPC catalyzes the carboxylation of PEP to oxaloacetate, which may be successively reduced to malate via cytosolic MDH; malate could be transported into the mitochondria via the dicarboxylic acid shuttle and converted to citrate by citrate synthase, as suggested by López-Millán et al. [20]. In agreement with these results, Rabotti et al. [22] reported that the accumulation of organic acids in Fe-deficient roots was also associated with an increased activity of some enzymes related to organic acid metabolism, such as MDH. As well, findings of M'sehli et al. [67, 96] showed that, the enhancement of organic acid accumulation in

Medicago roots under Fe deficiency was associated with an increase in MDH activity other than the PEPC activity. In addition, as shown by immunoblotting analysis, the enhancement of PEPC activity was attributable to an increase in protein expression, as previously found in cucumber [17] and in sugar beet [51]. The greatest increase in the PEPC activity frequently occurring upon addition of bicarbonate and lime to the growing medium, could be explained by the fact that PEPC catalyses the incorporation of bicarbonate into a C3 organic acid, PEP, producing oxaloacetate. Since bicarbonate has long been considered the major causal factor of Fe deficiency chlorosis in calcareous soils, the HCO_3^- fixing enzyme, PEPC, has been proposed as a component of adaptive strategies of plants to cope with poor external Fe availability in calcareous soils [97].

When plants are grown under low Fe concentration, the nutrient solutions may appear yellow. The presence of a yellow pigment in the nutrient solution of Fe-deficient plants was confirmed for tobacco [98], sugar beet [99], the desert shrub *Franseria dumosa* [100], sunflower [101], pumpkin [102], pepper [103] and lettuce [104]. The spectral characteristics of these yellow solution indicated that the colour was caused by flavin compounds. It has been assumed that the flavin excreted in the nutrient solution was Riboflavin (Rbfl), even if other forms, e.g. Rbfl 3'- and 5'-sulphate, can accumulate in the sub-apical zone of the root when grown at alkaline pH [105]. The exact role of flavins in Fe deficiency response is still unknown and it has been hypothesized that flavin accumulation in the roots may be an integral part of the Fe-reducing system of Strategy I plants. This hypothesis is based on the same localization of flavins accumulation and Fe reduction in the sub-apical roots and on the fact that the Fe reductase (FC-R) is a flavin-containing protein. However, at low pH these compounds can also be secreted in the nutrient solution and mediate extracellular electron transfer between FC-R and Fe deposits in the soil. The flavins exuded in the medium could also act as a plant-generated signal that could indirectly influence the rhizospheric microbial populations affecting Fe availability. To sustain the importance of flavins in response to Fe deficiency, a recent paper by Rellán-Álvarez et al. [33] showed that the largest change found in the proteome of root tip extracts from sugar beet plant grown under Fe deficiency corresponded to 6,7-dimethyl-8-ribityllumazine (DMRL) synthase. This enzyme catalyses the fourth step of Rbfl biosynthesis and Rbfl is the precursor of Rbfl sulphates, FMN and FAD, the last one being a cofactor for the root plasma membrane Fe reductase. Furthermore, it has been shown in Fe-deficient cucumber roots an increase in an old yellow enzyme-like protein (OYE) that it the first enzyme shown to contain flavin as a cofactor [32]. Proteins from OYE family can use either NADPH, NADH or both, thus classifying them as NAD(P)H oxidoreductase.

A common consequence of Fe deficiency is the increased production of reactive oxygen species (ROS). Physiological levels of ROS are important for cellular function such as signal transduction [106], however ROS overproduction may cause cellular damages to biomolecules and cellular structures such as DNA alteration, oxidation of proteins and lipid peroxidation [107]. Recently, several studies have explored the role of secondary metabolic pathways in plant response to oxidative stress.

The relationships between Fe deficiency and secondary oxidative stress remain controversial because Fe is either a constituent or a cofactor of many antioxidant enzymes and, at the same time it can act as a prooxidant through the Fenton reaction [108] (Figure 5).

As an enzyme constituent Fe is part of catalase (CAT), non-specific peroxidases (POD), ascorbate peroxidase (APX) and Fe superoxide dismutase (Fe-SOD).

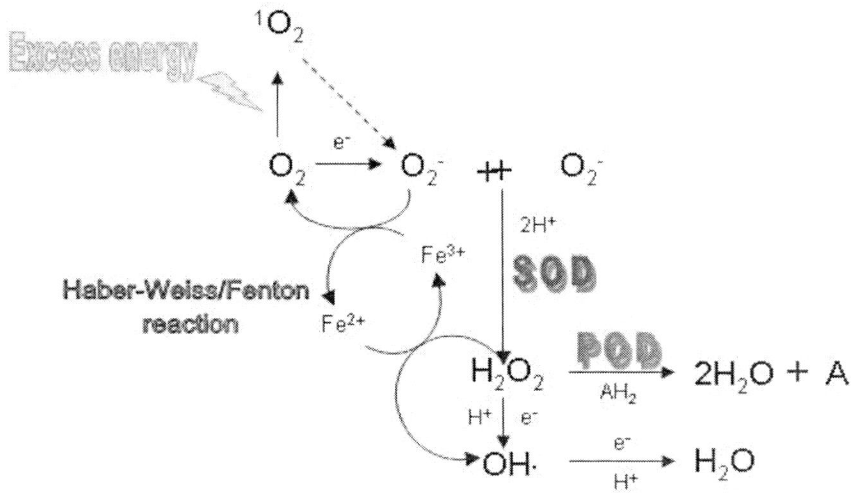

Figure 5. Interconversion of reactive oxygen species (ROS) derived from O_2. Fe ions that are mainly present in the oxidized form (Fe^{3+}) are reduced in the presence of O_2^- and, consequently, may catalyse the conversion of H_2O_2 to OH· by the Fenton or Haber-Weiss reactions. SOD: superoxide dismutase; POD: peroxidise.

Superoxide radical (O_2^-) is produced at any location where an electron transfer is present and thus in every compartment of the cell. Superoxide dismutases, converting O_2^- to H_2O_2, constitute the first line of defence against ROS in different plant species under several stress conditions [109]. Studies on plants grown in Fe-deprived conditions showed high SOD activity, mainly due to increased Cu/Zn or Mn-SOD isoforms [110, 111]. Recently, Donnini et al. [112] showed that total SOD activity was induced in Fe-deficient roots of both quince (BA29) and pear (cv. Conference), associated with Cu/Zn-SOD and Mn-SOD isoforms. However, this SOD induction appears not to be sufficient to detoxify O_2^-, which seems to be accumulated in the root tissues. Moreover, in BA29, which appear chlorotic under bicarbonate treatment, no increase in total SOD activity was detected, suggesting that the presence of bicarbonate could induce in this susceptible genotype a loss of O_2^- detoxification activity.

In addition to SOD activity, the intracellular level of H_2O_2 is controlled by other enzymes, the most important being CAT and PODs. Peroxidases, by means of their hydroxylic or peroxidative activity, can regulate both ROS production and scavenging in numerous cell compartments and thus they can be involved in many plant processes, such as growth and biotic/abiotic stress responses [113]. In the cell wall, PODs are present as soluble, ionically and covalently bound forms and they can catalyse cross-linking reactions, building a rigid cell wall, or produce ROS-generating wall-loosening reactions, to make it more flexible [114]. Additionally, PODs are enzymes directly involved in lignin biosynthesis by assembling lignin units through oxidative polymerization [114]. Several works have well documented that some growth conditions are responsible for the increase in cell-wall lignification which, by reducing cell growth, may represent a plant's adaptation to adverse conditions [115, 116]. With regard to plants grown under Fe deficiency, POD isoforms are differently affected. Ranieri et al. [117] showed, in Fe-deficient sunflower, a preferential reduction in the activity of those isoforms involved in H_2O_2 detoxification, rather than in the maintenance of cell-wall structure. Molassiotis et al. [111] showed that increased POD activity may be an important attribute linked to chlorosis tolerance in peach rootstocks. Interestingly, Donnini et al. [112] assayed POD activity using dianisidine, which is an aspecific substrate, and syringaldazine, a specific substrate for PODs involved in lignification. This led to the identification of a different effect of bicarbonate on genotypes differently susceptible to Fe chlorosis: while in the tolerant cv. Conference dian-POD was enhanced, suggesting that this treatment induced an increase in H_2O_2 scavenging, in BA29 the syr-POD undergoes an increase, playing a role in lignification by influencing cell-wall plasticity. While under several stress, root lignification could be implicated in the mechanism responsible for plant tolerance, under Fe deficiency, it could further impair mineral nutrition generating in quince higher susceptibility to this constraint.

In addition to antioxidative enzymes plants also synthesize antioxidative metabolites such as phenolic acids, glutathione and ascorbate.

Ascorbate (Asc) oxidation leads mainly to the formation of ascorbate free radical (AFR) [118]. Reductive mechanisms for Asc regeneration using b-type cytochrome or reduced ferredoxin as electron donors, have been identified both in PM and thylakoids [119, 120]. AFR can be also reduced to Asc by the enzyme monodehydroascorbate reductase (AFR-R), and its presence in leaves may indicate oxidative stress [119]. If not reduced, AFR disproportionates to Asc and dehydroascorbate, which is reduced to Asc by dehydroascorbate reductase using reduced glutathione (GSH) as electron donor [121].

GSH is a component of the Asc-glutathione cycle [122]. GSH and the GSSG ratio may operate as intracellular signalling mechanism in response to various stress [123]. The key enzyme for maintaining the GSH pool in a reduced state is the glutathione reductase (GR), a disulfide oxide reductase flavoprotein, dependent on NADPH as electron donor. In response to abiotic stresses the levels of Asc and GSH are generally increased and this may lead to enhanced stress tolerance in plant [123]. However their change during mineral deficiencies is scarcely studied.

Zaharieva et al. [124] showed in cucumber plants grown under Fe deficiency an enhanced level of both Asc and AFR-R activity, suggesting that this redox system could be activated under this stress condition. The same authors [125] suggested that in sugar beet, along with the membrane-bound FC-R reduction system, an additional Asc-mediated system could be also involved in Fe reduction and its activation could be part of the Strategy I responses. In the same roots, the concentration of GSH was enhanced together with GR activity, whereas the concentration of GSSG remained unchanged. However, in sugar beet roots the concentrations of GSH was10-fold lower than that of Asc then, its possible implication in Fe reduction process was rejected.

CONCLUSION

The efficiency of a plant response to Fe deprivation in its natural environment should be determined by its capacity to activate several mechanisms, which are a whole contribute to solving the problem. The more a plant will be able to mobilise Fe, the more it will be efficient. It appears that Fe acquisition under limiting conditions is not simply linked to the induction of the FC-R and of high affinity transporters, but the whole metabolism is subjected to a complex reprogramming. In order to both limits the effect of Fe lack and allows Fe uptake, both primary and secondary metabolisms undergo to a particular regulation. Indeed, while mitochondria reorganise its own metabolism avoiding the collapse, the others pathways, belonging either to the primary and secondary metabolism, activate all possible strategy to overcame at the same time energy demand, carbon skeleton production, turnover of reducing power and Fe acquisition. In this chapter we have proposed an overview of the complex regulation of metabolic events which are involved in the response to Fe deficiency in Strategy I plants. Despite the increased findings obtained until now, we are still far from gaining a full comprehension of the biochemical mechanisms involved. The new tools offered by proteomic and molecular approach will be helpful in the elucidation of the key regulatory points.

REFERENCES

[1] Maschner, H. *Mineral Nutrition of higher plants*. London: Academic press Ltd; 2 1995.

[2] Schmidt, W. (1999). Mechanism and regulation of reduction-based iron uptake in plants. *New Phytologist, 141,* 1-26.

[3] Curie, C. and Briat, J.F. (2003). Iron transport and signalling in plants. *Annual Review Plant Biology, 54,* 183-206.

[4] Rabotti, G. and Zocchi, G. (1994). Plasma membrane-bound H+-ATPase and reductase activities in Fe-deficient cucumber roots. *Physiologia Plantarum, 90,* 779-785.

[5] Dell'Orto, M., Santi, S., De Nisi, P., Cesco, S., Varanini, Z., Zocchi, G., Pinton, R. (2000). Development of Fe deficiency responses in cucumber (*Cucumis sativus* L.) roots: involvement of plasma membrane H^+-ATPase activity. *Journal of Experimental Botany, 51*, 695-701.

[6] Robinson, N.J., Procter, C.M., Connolly, E.L., Guerinot, M.L. (1999) A ferric-chelate reductase for iron uptake from soils. *Nature. 397,* 694-697.

[7] Eide, D.J., Broderius, M., Fett, J., Guerinot, M.L. (1996). A novel iron-regulated metal transporter from plants identified by functional expression in yeast. *Proceeings of the Nationa. Academy of Science USA. 93,* 5624-5628.

[8] Eckhardt, U., Mas Marques, A., Buckhout, T.J. Two iron-regulated cation transporters from tomato complement metal uptake-deficient yeast mutants, *Plant Molecular Biology* 2001 45, 437-448.

[9] Waters, B.M., Blevins, D.G., Eide, D.J. (2002). Characterization of FRO1, a pea ferricchelate reductase involved in root iron acquisition. *Plant Physiology, 129,* 85-94.

[10] Waters, B.M., Lucena, C., Romera, F.J., Jester, G.G., Wynn, A.N., Rojas, C.L., Alcantara, E., Perez-Vicente, R. (2007). Ethylene involvement in the regulation of H +-ATPase CsHA1 gene and of the new isolated ferric reductase CsFRO1 and iron transporter CsIRT1 genes in cucumber plants. *Plant Physiology and Biochemistry, 45,* 293-301.

[11] Santi, S., Cesco, S., Varanini, Z., Pinton, R. (2005) Two plasma membrane H+-ATPase genes are differentially expressed in iron-deficient cucumber plants. *Plant Physiology and Biochemistry, 43,* 285-292.

[12] Curie, C., Panaviene, Z.. Loulergue, C., Dellaporta, S.L., Briat, J.F., Walker, E.L. (2001) Maize *yellow stripe1* encodes a membrane protein directly involved in Fe(III) uptake. *Nature, 409,* 346–349.

[13] von Wiren, N., Klair, S., Bansal, S., Briat, J.F. Khodr, H., Shioiri, T., Leigh, R.A., Hider, R.C. (1999). Nicotianamine chelates both FeIII and FeII. Implications for metal transport in plants. *Plant Physiology, 119,* 1107–1114.

[14] Sijmons, P.C., and Bienfait, H.F. (1983) Source of electrons for extracellular Fe(III) reduction in iron-deficient bean plants. *Physiologia Plantarum,* 59, 409-415.

[15] Pontiggia, A., De Nisi, P., Zocchi, G. (2003). Effect of iron deficiency on RNA and protein synthesis in cucumber roots. *Journal of Plant Nutrition, 10-11,* 2177-2186.

[16] Schmidt, A., and Buckhout, T.J. (1997) The response of tomato roots (*Lycopersicon esculentum* Mill.) to iron deficiency stress: alterations in the pattern of protein synthesis. *Journal of Experimental Botany, 48,* 1909-1918.

[17] De Nisi, P., and Zocchi, G. (2000) Phoephο*enol*pyruvate carboxylase in cucumber (*Cucumis sativus* L.) roots under iron deficiency: activity and kinetic characterization. *Journal of Experimental Botany,* 51, 1903-1909.

[18] Connolly, E.L., Fett, J.P., Guerinot, M.L. (2002). Expression of the IRT1 metal transporter is controlled by metals at the levels of transcript and protein accumulation. *Plant Cell, 14,* 1347-1357.

[19] Vert, G.A., Briat, J.F., Curie, C. (2003). Dual regulation of the *Arabidopsis* high-affinity root iron uptake system by local and long-distance signals, *Plant Physiology, 132,* 796-804.

[20] López-Millán, A.F., Morales, F., Andaluz, S., Gogorcena, Y., Abadía, A., de Las Rivas, J., Abadía, J. (2000). Responses of sugar beet roots to iron deficiency. Changes in carbon assimilation and oxygen use. *Plant Physiology, 124,* 885-897.

[21] Herbik, A., Giritch, A., Horstmann, C., Becker, R., Balzer, H.J., Bäumlein, H., Stephan, U. (1996). Iron and copper nutrition-dependent changes in protein expression in a tomato wild type and the nicotianamine-free mutant *chloronerva*. *Plant Physiology, 111,* 533-540.

[22] Rabotti, G., De Nisi, P., Zocchi, G. (1995). Metabolic implications in the biochemical responses to iron deficiency in cucumber (*Cucumis sativus* L.) roots. *Plant Physiology, 107,* 1195-1199.

[23] Espen, L., Dell'Orto, M., De Nisi, P., Zocchi, G. (2000). Metabolic responses in cucumber (*Cucumis sativus* L.) roots under Fe-deficiency: a 31P-nuclear magnetic resonance *in vivo* study. *Planta, 210,* 985-992.

[24] Landsberg, E.C. (1994). Transfer cell formation in sugar beet roots induced by latent Fe Deficiency. *Plant and Soil, 165,* 197-205.

[25] Dell'Orto, M., Pirovano, L., Villalba, J.M., Gonzalez-Reyes, J.A., Zocchi, G. (2002). Localization of the plasma membrane H+-ATPase in Fe-deficient cucumber roots by immunodetection. *Plant and Soil, 241,* 11-17.

[26] Sijmons, P.C., Van Den Briel, W., Bienfait, H.F. (1984). Cytosolic NADPH is the electron donor for extracellular FeIII reduction in iron-deficient bean roots. *Plant Physiology, 75,* 219-221.

[27] Schmidt, W., and Schuck, C. (1996). Pyridine nucleotide pool size changes in iron-deficient *Plantago lanceolata* roots during reduction of external oxidants, *Physiologia. Plantarum, 98,* 215- 221.

[28] Zocchi, G. Metabolic changes in iron-stressed dicotyledonous plants. In: Barton LL, Abadía J. eds. Iron Nutrition in Plants and Rhizospheric Microorganisms. Dordrecht, The Netherlands: Springer 2006; 359-370.

[29] Thimm, O., Essigmann, B., Kloska, S., Altmann, T., Buckhout, T.J. (2001). Response of *Arabidopsis* to iron deficiency stress as revealed by microarray analysis. *Plant Physiology, 127,* 1030–1043.

[30] De Vos, C.R., Lubberding, H.J., Bienfait, H.F. (1986). Rhizosphere acidification as a response to iron deficiency in bean plants. *Plant Physiology, 81,* 842-846.

[31] Lucena, C., Waters, B.M., Romera, F.J., Garcia, M.J., Morales, M., Alcantara, E., Perez-Vicente, R. (2006). Ethylene could influence ferric reductase, iron trasposter and H^+-ATPase gene expression by affecting FER (or FER-like) gene activity. *Journal of Experimental Botany, 57,* 4145-4154.

[32] Donnini, S., Prinsi, B., Negri, A.S., Vigani, G., Espen, L., Zocchi, G. (2010). Proteomic characterization of iron deficiency responses in *Cucumis sativus* L. roots. *BMC Plant Biology, 10,* 268.

[33] Rellán-Álvarez, R., Andaluz, S., Rodríguez-Celma, J., Wohlgrmuth, G., Zocchi, G., Álvarez-Fernández, A., Fiehn, O., López-Millán, A.F., Abadía, J. (2010). Changes in the proteomic and metabolic profiles of Beta vulgaris root tips in response to iron deficiency and resupply. *BMC Plant Biology, 10,* 120-134.

[34] Li, J., Wu, X., Hao, S., Wang, X., Ling, H. (2008). Proteomic response to iron deficiency in tomato root. *Proteomics, 8,* 2299-311.

[35] Römheld, V., and Marschner, H. (1986). Mobilization of iron in the rhizosphere of different plant species. *Advanced Plant Nutrition, 2,* 155-204.

[36] Zocchi, G., and Cocucci, S.M. (1990). Fe uptake mechanism in Fe-efficient cucumber roots. *Plant Physiology, 92,* 908-911.

[37] De Nisi, P., Vigani, G., Zocchi, G. (2010). Modulation of iron responsive gene expression and enzymatic activities in response to changes of the iron nutritional status in *Cucumis sativus* L.. *Available from Nature Precedings.* <http://dx.doi.org/10.1038/npre.2010.4658.1>

[38] Davies, D.D. (1973). Control of and by pH. *Symposia of the Societ for Experimenta Biology. 27,* 513-520.

[39] Abadía, J., López-Millán, A.F., Rombolà, A., Abadía, A. (2002). Organic acids and Fe deficiency: a review. *Plant and Soil, 241,* 75-86.

[40] Day, D.A. *Plant Mitochondria: from genome to function.* Harvey millar and James Whelan (eds), 1-12, 2004.

[41] Vigani, G., Maffi, D., Zocchi, G. (2009). Iron availability affects the function of mitochondria in cucumber root. *New Phytologist, 182,* 127-136.

[42] Pascal, N., and Douce, R. (1993). Effect of iron deficiency on the respiration of sycamore (*Acer pseudoplatanus* L.) calls. *Plant Physiology, 103,* 1329–1338.

[43] Møller, I.M., and Lin, W. (1986). Membrane-bound NAD(P)H dehydrogenses in higher plant cells. *Annual Review of Plant Physiology, 37,* 309–334.

[44] Rasmusson, A.G., Heiser, V., Zabaleta, E., Brennicke, A., Grohmann, L. (1998). Physiological, biochemical and molecular aspects of mitochondrial complex I in plants. *Biochimica Biophysica Acta, 1364,* 101–111.

[45] Roberts, T.H., Fredlund, K.M., Møller, I.M. (1995). Direct evidence for the presence of two external NAD(P)H dehydrogenases coupled to the electron transport chain in plant mitochondria. *FEBS Letters, 373,* 307–309.

[46] Rasmusson, A.G., and Møller, I.M. (1991). Effect of calcium ions and inhibitors on internal NAD(P)H dehydrogenases in plant mitochondria. *European Journal of Biochemistry, 202,* 617–623.

[47] Melo, A.M.P., Roberts, T.H., Møller, I.M. (1996). Evidence for the presence of two rotenone-insensitive NAD(P)H dehydrogenases on the inner surface of the inner membrane of potato tuber mitochondria. *Biochimica and Biophysica Acta, 1276,* 133–139.

[48] Rasmusson, A.G., and Møller, I.M. (1991). NAD(P)H dehydrogenases on the inner surface of the inner mitochondrial membrane studied using inside-out submitochondrial particles. *Physiologia Plantarum, 83,* 357–365.

[49] Vigani, G., and Zocchi, G. (2010). Effect of Fe deficiency on mitochondrial alternative NAD(P)H dehydrogenases in cucumber roots. *Journal of Plant Physiology, 167,* 666-669.

[50] Lan, P., Li, W., Wen, T.N., Shiau, J.Y., Wu, Y.C., Lin, W., Schmidt, W. (2011). iTRAQ protein profile analysis of *Arabidopsis* roots reveals new aspects critical for iron homeostasis. *Plant Physiology, 155,* 821-834.

[51] Andaluz, S., López-Millán, A.F., Peleato, M,L., Abadía, J., Abadía, A. (2002). Increases of phospho*enol*pyruvate carboxylase activity in iron–deficient sugar beet roots: analysis of spatial localization and post-translational modification. *Plant and Soil, 241,* 43-48.

[52] López-Millán, A.F., Morales, F., Abadia, A., Abadia, J. (2000). Effects of iron deficiency on the omposition of the leaf apoplastic fluid and xylem sap in sugar beet. Implications for iron and carbon transpost. *Plant Physiology, 124,* 873-884.

[53] Larbi, A., Morales, F., Abadia, A., Abadia, J. (2001). Changes induced by Fe deficiency and Fe supply in the organic acid metabolism fluid of iron-deficient (*Beta vulgaris*) leaves. *Physiologia Plantarum, 112,* 31-38.

[54] López-Millán, A.F., Morales, F., Gogorcena, Y., Abadia, A., Abadia, J. (2009). Metabolic responses in iron deficienct tomato plants. *Journal of Plant Physiology, 166,* 375:384.

[55] Tiffin, L.O. (1966). Iron translocation I. plant culture, exudate sampling, iron-citrate analysis. *Plant Physiology, 41,* 510–514.

[56] Landsberg, E.C. (1986). Function of rhizodermal transfer cells in the Fe stress response mechanism of *Capsicum annuum* L.. *Plant Phisiology, 82,* 511-517.

[57] Dell'Orto, M., Pirovano, L., Villalba, J.M., Gonzalez-Reyes, J.A., Zocchi, G. (2002) Localization of the plasma membrane H^+-ATPase in Fe-deficient cucumber roots by immunodetection. *Plant and Soil 241,* 11–17.

[58] Logan, D.C., Scott, I., Tobin, A.K. (2004). ADL2a, like ADL2b, is involved in the control of higher plant mitochondrial morphology. *Journal of Experimental Botany, 55,* 783-785.

[59] Logan, D.C. (2006). The mitochondrial compartment. *Journal of experimental botany, 57,* 1225-1243.

[60] Bienfait, H.F. (1996). Is there a metabolic link between H^- excretion and ferric reduction by roots of Fe-deficient plant? A viewpoint. *Journal of Plant Nutrition, 19,* 105-129.

[61] Ebbighausen, H., Chen, J., Heldt, H.W. (1985). Oxaloacetate translocator in plant mitochondria. *Biochimica and Biophysica Acta 810,* 184–199.

[62] Journet, E.P., Neuburger, M., Douce, R. (1981). The role of glutamate oxaloacetate transaminase and malate dehydrogenase in the regeneration of NAD^+ for glycine oxidation by spinach leaf mitochondria. *Plant Physiology 67,* 467–469.

[63] Shen, W., Wei, Y., Dauk, M., Zheng, Z., Zou, J. (2003). Identification of a mitochondrial glycerol-3 phosphate dehydrogenase from *Arabidopsis thaliana*: evidence for a mitochondrial glycerol-3 phosphate shuttle in plants. *FEBS Lettere.* 536, 92-96.

[64] Shen, W., Wei, Y., Dauk, M., Tan, Y., Taylor, D.C., Selvaraj, G., Zuo, J. (2006). Involvement of a glycerol-3-phosphate dehydrogenase in modulating the NADH/NAD1 ratio provides evidence of a mitochondrial glycerol-3-phosphate shuttle in *Arabidopsis*. *Plant Cell 18,* 422-441.

[65] Welkie, G.W. (2000).Taxonomic distribution of dicotyledonous species capable of root excretion of riboflavin under iron deficiency. *Journal of Plant Nutrition*, *23*, 1819-1831.

[66] Jin, C.W., You, G.Y., He, Y.F., Tang, C., Wu, P., Zheng, S.J. (2007) Iron deficiency-induced secretion of phenolics facilitates the reutilization of root apoplastic iron in red clover. *Plant Physiology, 144*, 278-285.

[67] M'sehli, W., Youssfi, S., Donnini, S., Dell'Orto, M., De Nisi, P., Abdelly, C., Gharsalli, M. (2008) Root exudation and rhizosphere acidification by two lines of *Medicago ciliaris* in response to lime-induced iron deficiency. *Plant and Soil, 312,* 151–162.

[68] Olsen, R.A., Bennett, J.H., Blume, D., Brown, J.C. (1981) Chemical aspects of the Fe stress response mechanism in tomatoes. *Journal of Plant Nutrition, 3,* 905–921.

[69] Dell'Orto, M., De Nisi, P., Pontiggia, A., Zocchi, G. (2003) Fe deficiency responses in *Parietaria diffusa*: a calcicole plant. *Journal of Plant Nutrition, 26,* 2057-2068.

[70] Lambers, H., Cramer, M.D., Shane, M.W., Wouterlood, M., Poot, P., Veneklaas, E.J. (2003) Structure and functioning of cluster roots and plant responses to phosphate deficiency. *Plant and Soil,* 248, 43-59.

[71] Dakora, F.D. and Phillips, D.A. (2002) Root exudates as mediators of mineral acquisition in low-nutrient environments. *Plant and Soil, 245,* 35–47.

[72] Jin, C.W., You, G.Y., He, Y.F., Tang, C., Wu, P., Zheng, S.J. (2007) Iron deficiency-induced secretion of phenolics facilitates the reutilization of root apoplastic iron in red clover. *Plant Physiology, 144,* 278-285.

[73] Herms, D.A. and Mattson, W.J. (1992). The dilemma of plants: to grow or defend. *The Quarterly Review of Biology, 67,* 283-335.

[74] Lerdau, M. and Coley, P.D. (2002) Benefits of the carbon-nutrient balance hypothesis. *Oikos, 98,* 534-536.

[75] Herrmann, K.M. (1995). The shikimate pathway as an entry to aromatic secondary metabolism. *Plant Physiology, 107,* 2–7.

[76] Grace, S., Logan, B.A. (2000) Energy dissipation and radical scavenging by the plant phenylpropanoid pathway. *Philosophycal Transactions of the Royal Society of London, 355,* 1499–1510.

[77] Hahlbrock, K., Scheel, D. (1989). Physiology and molecular biology of phenylpropanoid metabolism. *Annual Review of Plant Physiology and Plant Molecular Biology, 40,* 347–369.

[78] Dixon, R.A., Paiva, N.L. (1995). Stress induced phenylpropanoid metabolism. *Plant Cell, 7,* 1085–1097.

[79] Beggs, C.J. and Wellman, E. Photocontrol of flavonoid biosynthesis. In: Kendrick RE, Kronenberg GHM (eds) *Photomorphogenesis in plants*. Dordrecht, the Netherlands; 1994;. 733–751.

[80] Solecka, D., Boudet, A.M., Kacperska, A. (1999). Phenylpropanoid anthocyanin changes in low-temperature treated oilseed rape leaves. *Plant Physiology and Biochemestry, 37,* 491–496.

[81] Trull, M.C., Guiltinan, M.J., Lynch, J.P., Deikman, J. (1997). The responses of wild-type and ABA mutant *Arabidopsis* thaliana plants to phosphorus starvation. *Plant, Cell and Environment, 20,* 85–92.

[82] Yamamoto, Y., Hachiya. A., Hamada, H., Matsumoto, H. (1998). Phenylpropanoids as a protectant of aluminium toxicity in cultured tobacco cells. *Plant and Cell Physiology, 39,* 950–957.

[83] Ohwaki, Y,, Sugahara, K. (1997). Active extrusion of protons and exudation of carboxylic acids in response to iron deficiency by roots of chickpea (*Cicer arietnum* L.). *Plant and Soil, 189,* 49–55.

[84] Welkie, G.W. (2000). Taxonomic distribution of dicotyledonous species capable of root excretion of riboflavin under iron deficiency. *Journal of Plant nutrition, 23,* 1819–1831.

[85] Nikolic, M. and Römheld, V., (1999). Mechanism of Fe uptake by leaf symplast: is Fe inactivation in leaf a cause of Fe deficiency chlorosis?. *Plant and Soil, 215,* 229–237.

[86] Tyler, G. and Ström, L. (1995). Differing organic acid exudation pattern explains calcifuge and acidifuge behaviour of plants. *Annals Botany,75,* 75–88.

[87] Jones, D.L. (1998). Organic acids in the rhizosphere – a critical review. *Plant and Soil, 205,* 25-44.

[88] Rengel, Z. and Römheld, V. (2000). Root exudation and Fe uptake and transport in wheat genotypes differing in tolerance to Zn deficiency. *Plant and Soil, 222,*25-34.

[89] Römheld, V., Awad, F. (2000) Significance of root exudates in aquisition of heavy metals from a contaminated calcareous soil by graminaceous species. *Jornal of Plant Nutrition, 23,* 1857-1866.

[90] Yang, C.-H., and Crowley, D. E. (2000). Rhizosphere microbial community structure in relation to root location and plant iron nutritional status. *Applied Environmental Microbiology, 66,* 345-351.

[91] Sun, L.Q., Zhang, H.Q., Li, Y.Y. (1987). Studies on dispersal of sterile *Carposina niponensis* using mark-release-recapture technique. *Acta Agriculturae Nucleatae Sinica, 1,*29-37.

[92] Rombolà, A., Mozzanti, F., Sorrenti, G., Marangoni, B. Plant water extracts: a new strategy to overcome Fe chlorosis in fruit trees. In: Book of Abstracts of the XXVIth International Horticultural Congress. Toronto, Canada; 2002

[93] Ollat, N., Laborde, B., Neveux, M., Diakou, V.P., Renaud, C., Moing, A. (2003). Organic acid metabolism in roots of various grapevine (vitis) rootstocks submitted to iron efficiency and bicarbonate nutrition. *Journal of Plant Nutrition, 26,* 2165–2176.

[94] Lambers, H., Juniper, D., Cawthray, G.R., Veneklaas, E.J., Martinez-Ferri, E. (2002). The pattern of carboxylate exudation in *Banksia grandis* (Proteaceae) is affected by the form of phosphate added to the soil. *Plant and Soil, 238,* 111–122.

[95] Veneklaas, E.J., Stevens, J., Cawthray, G.R., Turner, S., Grigg A.M., Lambers, H. (2003). Chickpea and white lupin rhizosphere carboxylates vary with soil properties and enhance phosphorus uptake. *Plant and Soil, 248,* 187–197.

[96] M'sehli, W., Dell'Orto, M., De Nisi, S., Donnini, S., Chedly, A., Zocchi, G., Gharsalli, M. (2009). Responses of two ecotypes of *Medicago ciliaris* to direct and bicarbonate-induced iron deficiency conditions. *Acta Physiologiae plantarum, 31,*667-673.

[97] Rombolà, A.D., Gogorcena, Y., Larbi, A., Morales, F., Baldi, E., Marangoni, B., Tagliavini, M., Abadia, J. (2005). Iron deficiency-induced changes in carbon fixation and leaf elemental composition of sugar beet (*Beta vulgaris*) plants. *Plant and Soil, 271,* 39–45.

[98] Welkie, G. W.; Miller, G. W. (1960). Iron nutrition of *Nicotiana tabacum L.* in relation to riboflavin, riboflavin-5-phosphate, and flavin adenine dinucleotide content. *Plant Physiology, 35(4),* 516– 520.

[99] Susín, S., Abián, J., Peleato, M., Sánchez-Baeza, F., Abadía, A., Gelpi, E., Abadía, J. (1994). Flavin excretion from roots of iron-deficient sugar beet (*Beta vulgaris L.*) *Planta, 193(4),* 514– 519.

[100] Wallace, A. Root excretions in tobacco plants and possible implications on the iron nutrition of higher plants. In: Wallace, A., Ed. *Regulation of the Micronutrients Status of Plants by Chelating Agents and Other Factors.* Los Angeles: A. Wallace Publ.; 1971; 136– 139.

[101] Venkat, R., Marschner, H., Römheld, V. (1972). Effect of iron nutritional status on iron uptake, substrate pH and production and release of organic acid and riboflavin by sunflower plants. *Z. Pflanzenernähr. Bodenk., 132,*177-190.

[102] Kannan, S. (1988). Physiological responses associated with Fe-deficiency stress in different plant species. *Journal of Plant Nutrition, 11,* 1185-1192.

[103] Welkie, G.M., Hekmat-Shoar, H., Miller, G.W., Responses of pepper plants to iron deficiency: solution pH and riboflavin. In: van Beusichem M.L. (Ed.) *Plant Nutrition-*

Physiology and Application. Kluwer Academic, Dordnecht, The Netherlands; 1990; 207–211.

[104] Welkie, G.W. and Miller, G. W. (1992). Iron stress and salt stress responses of lettuce (*Lactuca sativa* L.). *Journal of Plant Nutrition, 5(10)1,*1757-1764.

[105] Susín, S., Abián, J, Peleato, M.L., Sánchez-Baeza, F., Abadía, A., Gelpí, E. (1993). Riboflavin 3'- and 5'-sulfate, two novel flavins accumulating in the roots of iron-deficient sugar beet (*Beta vulgaris*). *The Journal of Biological Chemistry, 28*, 20958–20965.

[106] Smeets, K., Ruytinx, J., Semane, B., Van Belleghem, F., Remans, T., Van Sanden, S., Vangronsveld, J., Cuypers, A. (2008). Cadmium-induced transcriptional and enzymatic alterations related to oxidative stress. *Environmental of Experimental Botany, 63,* 1–8.

[107] De Vos, C.H.R., Vonk, M.J., Schat, H. (1992) Glutathione depletion due to copper induced phytochelatin synthesis causes oxidative stress in *Silene cucubalus*. *Plant Physiology, 98,* 853-858.

[108] Halliwell, B. and Gutteridge J. (1984). Oxygen toxicity, oxygen radicals, transition metals and disease. *Biochemical Journal, 219,* 1–14.

[109] Alscher, R.G., N. Erturk, Hearth, L.S. (2002). Role of superoxide dismutases (SODs) in controlling oxidative stress in plants. *Journal of Experimental Botany, 53,* 1331–1341.

[110] Iturbe-Ormaexte, I., Moran, J.F., Arrese-Igor, C., Gogorcena, Y., Klucas, R.V., Becana M. (1995). Activated oxygen and antioxidant defenses in iron deficient pea plants. *Plant, Cell and Environment, 18*, 421–429.

[111] Molassiotis, A., Tanou, G., Diamantidis, G., Patakas, A., Therios, I. (2006) Effects of 4-month Fe deficiency exposure on Fe reduction mechanism, photosynthetic gas exchange, chlorophyll fluorescence and antioxidant defense in two peach rootstocks differing in Fe deficiency tolerance. *Journal of Plant Physiology, 163,* 176–185.

[112] Donnini, S., Dell'Orto, M., Zocchi, G. (2011). Oxidative stress responses and root lignification induced by Fe deficiency conditions in pear and quince genotypes. *Tree physiology, 31,* 102-113.

[113] Passardi, F., Cosio, C., Penel, C., Dunand, C. (2005). Peroxidases have more functions than a Swiss army knife. *Plant Cell Reports, 24,* 255–265.

[114] Lewis, N.G. and Yamamoto, E. (1990). Lignin: occurrence, biogenesis and biodegradation. *Annual Review of Plant Physiology and Plant Molecular Biology, 41,* 455–496.

[115] Jbir, N., Chaïbi, W., Ammar, S., Jemmali, A., Ayadi, A. (2001). Root growth and lignification of two wheat species differing in their sensitivity to NaCl, in response to salt stress. *Comptes Rendus de l' Academie des Sciences : Series III Science de la Vie, 324,*863–868.

[116] Lee, B.R., Kim, K.Y., Jung, W.J., Avice, J.C., Ourry, A., Kim, T.H. (2007). Peroxidases and lignification in relation to the intensity of water-deficit stress in white clover (*Trifolium repens* L.). *Journal of Experimental Botany, 58,* 1271–1279.

[117] Ranieri, A., Castagna, A., Baldan, B., Soldatini, G.F. (2001). Iron deficiency differently affects peroxidase isoforms in sunflower. *Journal of Experimental Botany, 52,* 25–35.

[118] Arrigoni, O., Dipierro, S., Borraccino, G. (1981). Ascorbate free radical reductase a key enzyme of the ascorbic acid system. *FEBS letters, 125,* 242-245.

[119] Asada, K. The role of ascorbate peroxidase and monodehydroascorbate reductase in H_2O_2 scavenging in plants. In: Scandalios J.G. (ed.) *Oxidative stress and the molecular*

biology of antioxidant defenses. Cold Spring Harbor Laboratory Press, NY; 1997; 715-735.

[120] Horemans, N., Asard, H., Caubergs, R.J. (1994). The role of ascorbate free radical as an electron acceptor to cytochrome b-mediated trans-plasma membrane electron transfer in higher plants. *Plant Physiology, 104,*1455-1458.

[121] Noctor, G. and Foyer, C.H. (1998) Ascorbate and glutathione: keeping active oxygen under control. *Annual Review Plant Physiology Plant Molecular Biology, 49,* 249-279.

[122] Foyer, C.H., Lelandais M., Galap C., Kunert, K.J. (1991). Effects of elevated cytosolic glutathione reductase activity on the cellular gluthatione pool and photosynthesis in leaves under normal and stress conditions. *Plant Physiology, 97,* 863-872.

[123] Foyer, C.H., López-Delgrado, H., Dat, J.F., Scott, I.M. (1997). Hydrogen peroxide and glutathione-associated mechanisms of acclimatory stress tolerance and signalling. *Physiologia Plantarum, 100,* 241-254.

[124] Zaharieva, T., Yamashita, K., Matsumoto, H. (1999). Iron deficiency induced changes in ascorbate content and enzyme activities related to ascorbate metabolism in cucumber roots. *Plant and Cell Physiology, 40,* 273-280.

[125] Zaharieva, T. and Abadía, J. (2003). Iron deficiency enhances the levels of ascorbate, glutathione and related enzymes in sugar beet roots. *Protoplasma, 221,*269-275.

In: Iron Deficiency and Its Complications
Editor: Yildiz Dincer
ISBN 978-1-61324-854-6

Chapter 2

Iron Deficiency and Its Complications

Anu Maheshwari and Jagdish Chandra
Department of Pediatrics, Lady Hardinge Medical College, New Delhi

Introduction

Iron deficiency (ID) remains the most prevalent single-nutrient deficiency in developing and developed countries. The World Health Organization[1] estimates that, worldwide, 1.6- 2 billion people are anemic. Although ID is responsible for at least half of the cases of anemia, there are other possible causes, including genetic, infectious, and other nutritional deficiencies. It is estimated that when anemia prevalence reaches 20%, ID exists in 50% of the population, and when anemia prevalence exceeds 40%, the entire population suffers from some degree of ID.[2] Infants, children, and women of reproductive age are at highest risk of developing ID and iron deficiency anemia (IDA), largely because of their high physiological requirements associated with growth combined with greater losses and poor dietary intake. Globally, almost half of preschool-aged children and pregnant women and close to one-third of non-pregnant women have anemia [1, 2].

However, more important than anemia, the more common ID without anemia may adversely affect long-term neurodevelopment and behavior in children [3, 4].[4] Iron deficiency anemia also weakens the immune status and resistance to infections [5], lower work capacity [6], and to impair child growth [7]. Infants with anemia showed slower psychomotor and mental development, and many of these effects seem irreversible [8, 9]. Even ID without anemia affects cognition and motor development in children and adolescents as well [10, 11]. Association of iron deficiency with febrile seizures, pica, breath holding spells, restless leg syndrome and thrombosis is increasingly being recognized.

It is estimated that worldwide, 200 million children do not reach their full developmental potential because of preventable causes. ID was identified as one of the leading nutrition-related causes of impaired child development, along with stunting and iodine deficiency. Correction of ID is likely to contribute to better child development, particularly in geographical regions in which ID is endemic. With an estimated 187 million stunted children iron interventions alone will not alleviate all disparities [12]. Nevertheless, micronutrient interventions for children including iron fortification, were considered the most cost-effective solution for solving some of the world's biggest challenges, including malnutrition [13, 14].

DEFINITIONS

Anemia

A hemoglobin (Hb) concentration 2 SDs below the mean Hb concentration for a normal population of the same gender and age range, as defined by the World Health Organization, the United Nations Children's Fund, and United Nations University [15]. On the basis of the 1999–2002 US National Health and Nutrition Examination Survey, anemia is defined as a Hb concentration of less than 11.0 g/dL for both male and female children aged 12 through 35 months [16, 17]. For certain populations (ie, people living at high altitudes), adjustment of these values may be necessary.

Iron Deficiency

A state in which there is insufficient iron to maintain normal physiologic functions. ID results from inadequate iron absorption to accommodate an increase in requirements attributable to growth or resulting from a long-term negative iron balance. Either of these situations leads to a decrease in iron stores as measured by serum ferritin (SF) concentrations or bone marrow iron content. ID may or may not be accompanied by IDA.

Iron-Deficiency Anemia

An anemia (as defined above) that results from ID.

Recommended Dietary Allowance for Iron

The average daily dietary intake that is sufficient to meet the nutrient requirements of nearly all individuals (97%–98%) of a given age and gender.

Adequate Intake for Iron

This term is used when there is not enough information to establish a recommended dietary allowance for a population (eg, term infants, 0–6 months of age). The adequate intake is based on the estimated average nutrient intake by a group (or groups) of healthy individuals.

Iron Metabolism

Iron is a key element in the metabolism of all living organisms. Iron is a component of heme, which is the active site of electron transport in cytochromes and cytochrome oxygenase, essential coenzymes in the Krebs cycle. The heme moiety of hemoglobin and myoglobin binds O_2, providing the means to transfer O_2 from the lungs to tissues. Heme is also the active site of peroxidases that protect cells from oxidative injury by reducing peroxides to water. Neither bacteria nor nucleated cells can proliferate when the supply of iron is insufficient.

Distribution of Iron

Hemoglobin

Hemoglobin is 0.34 percent iron by weight, contains approximately 2 g of body iron in men and 1.5 g in women. One milliliter of packed erythrocytes contains approximately 1 mg of iron.

Storage Compartment

Iron is stored either as ferritin or as hemosiderin. The former is water-soluble; the latter is water-insoluble. Ferritin is found in virtually all cells of the body and also in tissue fluids. The plasma (serum) ferritin concentration usually correlates roughly with total-body iron stores, making measurement of serum ferritin levels important in the diagnosis of disorders of iron metabolism. Hemosiderin is found predominantly in macrophages. Hemosiderin contains approximately 25 to 30 percent iron by weight.

Myoglobin

Myoglobin is structurally similar to hemoglobin, but it is monomeric. It is present in small amounts in all skeletal and cardiac muscle cells, where it may serve as an oxygen reservoir to protect against cellular injury during periods of oxygen deprivation.

Tissue Iron Compartment

Tissue Iron Compartment normally amounts to 6 to 8 mg. This includes cytochromes and other iron-containing enzymes. Although a small compartment, it is an extremely vital one and is sensitive to iron deficiency.

Transport Compartment

From the standpoint of its total iron content, normally about 3 mg, the transport compartment of plasma is the smallest but the most active of the iron compartments: Its iron normally turns over at least 10 times each day.

Transferrins and Lactoferrins

Transferrins and Lactoferrins comprise a group of glycoproteins that transport iron in plasma and in milk, respectively. They are single polypeptide chains of approximately 80 kDa. Each molecule has two binding sites for Fe^{+++}.

PHYSIOLOGICAL CONSEQUENCES OF IRON DEFICIENCY

Erythrocyte Survival and Ferrokinetics

Slight to moderate shortening of erythrocyte survival is characteristic of iron-deficiency anemia, particularly when it is severe. The plasma iron transport rate may be normal or increased [18]. The percentage of iron utilized in hemoglobin synthesis is normal or increased. There is usually little or no evidence of ineffective erythropoiesis.

Iron-Containing Proteins

As the body becomes depleted of iron, changes occur in many tissues. Hemosiderin and ferritin virtually disappear from marrow and other storage sites. There is a decreased activity of many other important iron proteins: cytochrome c, cytochrome oxidase, succinic dehydrogenase, aconitase, xanthine oxidase, and myoglobin [19].

Muscular Function and Exercise Tolerance

Iron-deficient rats have impaired exercise tolerance and are prone to lactic acidosis when exercised. The activity of α-glycerophosphate dehydrogenase was diminished in the skeletal muscle of iron-deficient rats, and this finding might explain the greater proclivity of iron-deficient rats to lactic acidosis upon exercise [20, 21]. The brown fat of iron-deficient rats has lower-than-normal activities of the reduced form of nicotinamide adenine dinucleotide and of succinate and α-glycerophosphate oxidases [22]. Besides these metabolic aberrations of muscle cells in iron deficient rodents, ultrastructural studies show swollen mitochondria with distorted cristae, and there is evidence of mitochondrial DNA damage [23]. Despite these changes, mitochondrial cytochrome c increases adaptively on repetitive electrical stimulus of muscle [24]. In human athletes, iron supplementation has been associated with improved performance, [25-29] although earlier studies did not document any aberrations in oxygen consumption in exercising iron-deficient human subjects [30].

Neurologic Changes

Monoamine oxidase (MAO) activity is low in the liver and platelets of patients with iron deficiency. MAO is involved in the synthesis and catabolism of important neurotransmitters such as dopamine, norepinephrine, and serotonin. Furthermore, iron-deficient children and iron-deficient rats excrete substantially more urinary norepinephrine than do iron-replete children or rats, an anomaly that is corrected within a few days of inception of iron therapy [31]. The brains of iron-deficient rats exhibit reduction in the number of dopamine D2 receptors that are also important in neurotransmission.

Host Defenses

Iron deficiency affects immune function and the susceptibility to infection. Some studies found that iron depletion prevents growth of microorganisms and therefore protects against infections; others observed that iron deficiency impairs host defenses [32].

Growth and Metabolism

Iron-deficiency anemia is associated with reduction in children's height, and treatment promotes growth. Together with zinc deficiency, it has been held responsible for dwarfism.

Histologic Findings

Iron deficiency may lead to histologic changes in various organs. The rapidly proliferating cells of the upper part of the alimentary tract seem particularly susceptible to the effect of iron deficiency. There may be atrophy of the mucosa of the tongue and esophagus, stomach, and small intestine.

Buccal mucosa has shown thinning and keratinization of epithelium and increased mitotic activity. Widening of diploic spaces of bones, particularly those of the skull and hands, may be a consequence of chronic iron deficiency beginning in infancy. In the skull, this is of the same character as in thalassemia, except that in β-thalassemia major there is maxillary hypertrophy, whereas in severe iron-deficiency anemia maxillary growth and pneumatization are normal. The sella turcica may be abnormally small in iron-deficient children, and it has been suggested that this implies reduction in pituitary hormonal secretion in long-standing iron-deficiency anemia.

Complications of Iron Deficiency

Iron Deficiency and Development

Over the past 3 decades, substantial understanding of the relationship between ID and development or behavior in infants and young children has been developed. A conceptual framework for how ID may affect child development suggests that the relationship between iron and development may be direct, through an effect on brain function and structure, or indirect, through changes in exploratory behavior of the anemic child, which affects the quality of parent–child interactions.[33] These in turn indicate that there is strong evidence indicating that IDA is associated with poorer developmental ratings in infants [34] and with lower scores on cognitive function tests and educational achievement tests in children [35]. The negative effect of IDA on child development tends to be long lasting: children without anemia who had been iron deficient or anemic as infants had lower IQ scores at age 2–7 years than children who had not been anemic in the first year of life. In a follow-up study from Costa Rica, children who had been iron-deficient as infants scored persistently poorer on cognitive tests up to the age of 19 years, and these effects were greater in children from high-risk environments, suggesting an interaction between environment or social stimulation and ID [36].

New insights are emerging from recent and ongoing investigations into the role of iron in neurocognitive and neurobehavioral development. The uptake of iron through the blood–brain barrier appears to be regulated and dependent on iron status [37] such that there is a higher rate when iron status is low and a lower rate when it is high [37, 38]. In addition, this uptake process is highly selective and not reflective of overall blood–brain barrier permeability [37, 39]. The brain obtains iron primarily via Tf (transferrin) and Tf receptors expressed in endothelial cells on the brain microvasculature [37, 40]. ID affects neurogenesis and neurochemistry during brain development. Animal studies show structural impairments of the hippocampus in ID, whereas in the striatum, less arborization and fewer affected dendrites have been observed [41]. ID also results in a different location and impaired functioning of the oligodendrocytes in the rat brain, resulting in altered composition and amount of myelin in white matter [37, 42]. The role of iron in the production of hormones from the monoaminergic pathways, particularly dopamine and norepinephrine, illustrates the importance of iron in neurochemistry [37, 43-46]. The concentration of iron in the brain is highest at birth, decreases through weaning, and then begins to increase coincident with the onset of myelination and greater expression of transferrin mRNA. Noninvasive techniques are now available to measure developmental patterns of iron accumulation in the developing brain. Magnetic resonance imaging has been used to map iron distribution in the brains of children and adolescents [47, 48]. The deposition of iron in the brain varies according to region and age. Regions of the brain rich in iron in adulthood (e.g., the substantia nigra, globus pallidus) are not the regions that have a high iron content in early life, when the highest concentrations of iron are found in the globus pallidus, caudate nucleus, putamen, and substantia nigra [49]. In addition, regions of the brain that are rich in iron are not necessarily the ones that dietary ID most affects. It might be that the different regional needs for iron in the brain during different stages of neurodevelopment impart a differential sensitivity of brain regions to nutritional deprivation of iron. The effect of iron interventions may reverse the abnormalities in the affected brain regions depending on when in development the iron repletion occurs. In rats that had been on iron-deficient diets from mid-gestation onward, early iron treatment (at 4 days postpartum) normalized brain iron concentrations, monoamine concentrations, and monoamine transporter and receptor densities in most brain regions. Rats that had been exposed to gestational ID had lower dopamine transporter densities in caudate and substantia nigra than control animals, but these abnormalities were normalized after early iron repletion. In contrast, iron repletion later in life, at weaning, did not reverse the effect of gestational ID. These findings suggested the existence of a critical window of opportunity for reversing the detrimental effects of ID in utero on brain development, at least in rats and probably also in humans [50]. ID is also known to affect neurochemistry in the developing brain. ID during lactation in infant rats resulted in abnormal dopamine concentrations in the brain,[37] and these abnormalities in dopamine metabolism and in behaviors that depend on striatal dopamine function were not completely restored after aggressive iron therapy [51]. These findings strengthen the hypothesis that the sensitivity of a brain region to loss of iron during development is likely to be related to the regional development requirements for iron during that period.

The results of intervention trials studying the effect of iron treatment on cognitive and motor development scores in iron-deficient infants have been inconsistent. Four of six recent randomized controlled trials of iron supplementation in infancy that assessed social and emotional behavior found a benefit from iron,[52] but there were conflicting effects on cognitive performance tasks [35].

In children aged 2 years and older, iron treatment of iron deficient children with and without anemia led to better scores on cognitive function tests in six of eight trials [35, 53-55]. The differential effects of iron treatment on development in children according to age (<2 years versus ≥ 2 years) suggest the existence of a sensitive window in brain development during which environmental effects, such as ID, may be at least partly irreversible.

New emerging insights into the role of iron during brain development have allowed researchers to design intervention studies with sensitive measurements of child development, focusing on specific functions in areas of the brain known to be most sensitive to ID. The advantage of a combination of techniques, measuring responses in the brain and performance on cognitive tasks, enabled scientists to better define the role of iron in child development. Rocanglio et al. [56] found differences between the maturation of central conduction time of the auditory brain stem in infants who were anemic at 6 months of age and that of infants who were not anemic. At 12 and 18 months, the infants who were initially anemic showed longer conduction times than the infants who were not anemic, even though their iron status had been restored to normal and they were no longer anemic. Burden et al. [57] used event-related potential techniques to locate the corresponding brain areas involved during a delayed processing- information task in iron-deficient infants. In a delayed-processing-information task, iron-deficient infants aged 9–12 months were less able to distinguish a familiar face from a stranger's face than non-deficient infants, as confirmed according to event-related potential graphs, perhaps because of alterations in the striatum and hippocampus in the iron-deficient infants. Changes in the hippocampus are of particular interest because of the role of this region of brain in discrimination between novel and familiar stimuli in recognition memory. The role of iron in dopamine production allowed researchers to better design tests of the effect of ID on socio-emotional development by focusing on behaviors that are known to be regulated by dopamine. In a cohort study, 77 African American infants aged 9–10 months were tested on shyness, orientation and engagement, and response to unfamiliar pictures; the scores of iron sufficient infants for socio-emotional development were the highest, while those of iron-deficient infants with anemia were the worst, and those of iron-deficient infants without anemia were intermediate [58]. These findings are consistent with early disruption of the dopamine system, due to ID, and they contribute to a growing understanding that altered affect and response to novelty are among the core deficits in early ID [58].

Iron Deficiency and Febrile Seizures

Febrile seizures are defined by the National Institute of Health as "an event in infancy or childhood usually occurring between three months and five years of age, associated with fever but without evidence of intracranial infection or defined cause for the seizure [59]." They are the most common cause of convulsions in childhood, occurring in 2% to 4% of North American children [60]. The peak age of febrile seizures is 18 months, with recurrent episodes occurring in one third of patients [61]. Currently identified risk factors for febrile seizure include having a first- or second-degree relative with a history of febrile seizure, maternal smoking in pregnancy, low birth weight, neonatal stay of > 30 days, attendance at day care, increased number of febrile illnesses, fever greater than 39.4°C, and particular infectious illnesses [62].

Iron has been found to act as a cofactor in a number of enzymatic reactions at the cellular level, and it effects neurotransmitter production and function, hormone function, and DNA replication [63, 64]. The peak age for ID is between 1 and 2 years, which coincides with the peak incidence for febrile seizures. ID is also associated with neurological problems in young children, including developmental delay, stroke, breath-holding spells, and pseudo tumor cerebri [65].

Recently, four small studies have been published investigating a possible relationship between ID and febrile seizures, with varying results.[66-69] Three of the studies found that ID was associated with increased risk of febrile seizures,[67-69] whereas the fourth found that children with ID were less likely to have a febrile seizure.[66] Factors that may have contributed to these contrary results include small patient numbers and different diagnostic criteria for the diagnosis of ID in the setting of an illness. Hartfield et al published a retrospective case control study with 361 patients. They demonstrated that a total of 9% of cases had iron deficiency (ID) and 6% had iron deficiency anemia (IDA), compared to 5% and 4% of controls respectively and concluded that children with febrile seizures were almost twice as likely to be iron deficient as those with febrile illness alone [70].

Possible mechanisms include increased susceptibility of the developing brain to febrile and other seizures. Experimental evidence has also suggested that maturational changes of both inhibitory and excitatory neurotransmitters and other mechanisms influence the developing brain's susceptibility to seizure activity [61, 62]. Role of viral infection in the etiology of febrile seizures also has been postulated. Underlying mechanisms include the generation of fever, or an elevated/inappropriate response to cytokines generated in association with infection [71]. With advances in molecular genetics, there are also attempts at identifying causative genetic mutations in family groupings responsible for febrile seizures [72]. One may therefore hypothesize that the disruption of normal neurotransmitter activity caused by ID may be the mechanism that predisposes children with ID to febrile seizures.

Iron Deficiency and Breath-Holding Spells

Breath-holding episodes have also been associated with iron deficiency. These benign episodes occur in up to 27% of children [73, 74]. Although benign in nature, breath-holding episodes result in much parental anxiety. The pathophysiology is unclear, although autonomic dysregulation resulting in vagally mediated cardiac arrest and subsequent cerebral anoxia has been proposed [74, 75]. Anemia has been suggested to exacerbate the likelihood of breath-holding episodes because the lower hemoglobin results in more rapid cerebral anoxia secondary to decreased oxygen-carrying capacity [73, 76]. Also, iron-deficient children are more irritable, which increases the likelihood of a spell [73].

It is not known whether, or if so how, iron deficiency leads to breath-holding attacks. Iron deficiency anemia may lead to adverse effects on oxygen uptake in the lungs and therefore reduces available oxygen to the tissues, including central nervous system tissue [76, 77]. Not all children with breath-holding attacks are iron deficient at baseline [74, 78]. The majority of studies classify children as being iron deficient on the basis of low hematological indices such as hemoglobin, serum transferrin, mean corpuscular hemoglobin (MCH) and mean corpuscular volume (MCV) without any evidence of bone marrow failure. Values below the normal range signify iron deficiency anemia. It is unclear why iron-replete children may respond to iron therapy for breath-holding attacks. It is possible that iron supplementation maximizes neurotransmitter synthesis and function. Iron has a role in catecholamine metabolism and the functioning of enzymes and neurotransmitters in the central nervous system [79]. The resolution of attacks during treatment with iron may be related to the functional restoration of these neurotransmitters.

It has been hypothesized that the clinical and hematological picture of breath-holding attacks relates to the interactions of cerebral erythropoietin (EPO), nitric oxide and interleukin-1 [78, 80]. It has been suggested that "increased brain erythropoietin production has a protective effect during breath-holding attacks, but where this does not compensate for the severity of anoxic attacks, tonic-clonic movements may develop". In addition, it has been postulated that the enhanced erythropoiesis resulting from increased EPO secretion during hypoxia can also induce at least a temporary state of iron-deficient erythropoiesis in iron-replete patients [78]. Repeated breath-holding attacks cause episodes of hypoxia, including cerebral anoxia. Short-lived tonic-clonic movements of the limbs may occur as a result of the cerebral anoxia. A further and protective response to cerebral anoxia is for brain EPO production to increase. As iron is consumed in erythropoiesis, a relative deficiency of iron stores occurs. Over time the child may become anemic and exhibit behavioral 'irritability', leading to further breath-holding attacks. This theory may also explain why breath-holding attacks occur in non-anemic children, as there is a relative deficiency of iron stores and distribution rather than a depletion of the total amount of body iron.

In the Daoud study [74], of the 33 children treated with iron 17 children had complete resolution of breath-holding attacks (BHA) and 12 displayed partial remission; iron had no effect on the frequency of breath holding in four children. Of the 34 children treated with placebo, only two had partial remission of BHAs. No child in the control group had complete remission of BHAs. The study found a 14-fold, significant reduction ($P < 0.01$) in the frequency of BHAs (88%) in the treatment group compared with the 6% frequency in the placebo group. Iron supplementation was of particular benefit in children with BHAs who have iron deficiency anemia, with the response being predicted by and correlating to improvements in hemoglobin values.

Holowach et al. [75] demonstrated a correlation between breath-holding episodes and anemia in a retrospective study. One-hundred and sixty children 3 months to 3 years of age with breath-holding episodes were reviewed over a 10-year period. Two control groups were used, including one group of 192 children with febrile seizures or myoclonus and a group of 572 hospitalized children with other medical conditions. Hemoglobin values were compared between the groups. Of those with breath-holding episodes, 23.5% had hemoglobin concentrations less than 79 gm/L compared with 2.6% of the children with seizures and 6.9% of other hospitalized children. Other researchers have also demonstrated an association between iron deficiency anemia and breath-holding episodes with a decrease or resolution of the episodes after iron therapy [73, 81].

Cochrane review studied the effect of iron supplementation on the frequency and severity of breath-holding attacks in children. Iron supplementation (at 5 mg/kg/day of elemental iron for 16 weeks) reduced the frequency (number over time) or severity (measured as loss of consciousness or convulsive movements) of breath-holding attacks (BHAs) in children.

Iron Deficiency and Pseudo Tumor Cerebri

Since the 1800s, pseudo tumor cerebri secondary to iron deficiency has been a recognized phenomenon [83-89]. It is most common in young females [73-88]. The mechanism by which this occurs is unclear, although one theory suggests that tissue hypoxia leads to increased capillary permeability and primary brain edema, after which subsequent papilledema as a result of the increased intracranial pressure occurs [82, 88]. Other researchers have suggested that abnormalities in hemodynamics result in increased cerebral blood flow, causing increased intracranial pressure and papilledema [85, 88]. Also depletion of iron-containing enzymes has also been hypothesized to play a role [83, 86, 88]. In infancy, these changes may manifest as a bulging fontanel rather than papilledema [85]. Pseudo tumor cerebri in this setting is reversible with iron therapy.

Another neurologic abnormality observed with iron deficiency anemia is bilateral VI cranial nerve palsy. This is proposed to be a consequence of increased intracranial pressure or focal pontine ischemia [82].

Iron Deficiency and Thromboembolic Events

In Romeo and Juliet, Capulet screams at his daughter Juliet, ''Out, you greensickness carrion,'' when she refuses to marry the man he has chosen for her. Shakespeare was probably referring to a malady believed to occur commonly in young women: 'green-sickness' or 'chlorosis' which was later found to be a severe form of iron deficiency anemia which led to a greenish pallor of the skin, gastrointestinal complaints, growth retardation and amenorrhea [89, 90]. As early as 1861, von Dusch lists chlorosis as a cause of 'marantic' cerebral venous thrombosis (CVT) in his review on CVT [91]. The postmortem statistics of the University of Munich from 1888 to 1897 observed 460 'marantic', i.e. non-infectious thromboses of unknown origin, in 8578 cases. In 22 cases of 'marantic' CVT, 13% were thought to be caused by chlorosis [92]. Four years later, in 1899, Leichtenstern reviewed 86 cases of chlorotic venous thrombosis, of whom 35% suffered CVT [93]. By then, chlorosis was generally accepted as a risk factor for venous thrombosis in general, and CVT in particular. However, in the early 20th century chlorosis virtually disappeared as a disease entity. Since then, several case reports linked iron deficiency anemia with the onset of stroke or CVT. However, it is still unclear whether this is a chance association or a causal link. Secondary thrombocytosis has been implicated in many cases. Indeed, iron deficiency is a cause of reactive thrombocytosis, usually mild [94]. For instance, within a study group of children with iron deficiency, reactive thrombocytosis was found in up to one-third of them [95].

Nagai et al. [96] reported a case of severe iron deficiency with marked thrombocytosis ($1{,}020 \times 10^9$/l) that was complicated by central retinal vein occlusion. By contrast, Kinoshita et al. [97] described two cases of cerebral venous sinus thrombosis associated with iron deficiency and normal platelet count. Hartfield et al. [98] reported six children with iron deficiency who developed an ischemic stroke or venous thrombosis. Four of them had a concomitant thrombocytosis. In a prospective case–control study, Stolz et al. [99] found that severe anemia, along with thrombophilia and hypercholesterolemia, were independent risk factors for cerebral venous thrombosis.

The mechanisms causing reactive thrombocytosis in iron deficiency anemia are not completely understood. Iron is an important regulator of thrombopoiesis [100, 101]. Normal iron levels are required to prevent thrombocytosis by inhibiting thrombopoiesis, a minimum amount of iron is required to maintain platelet production. Thus, while thrombocytosis is usually associated with a mild iron deficiency and is the result of a lack of inhibition of thrombopoiesis, a severe defect of this metal may be accompanied by thrombocytopenia. However, studies on thrombopoietic cytokines failed to show any effect on reactive thrombocytosis in iron deficiency [94]. For instance, Akan et al. [102] assayed the serum levels of thrombopoietin, erythropoietin, leukemia inhibitor factor, IL-6, and IL-11 in patients with iron-deficient anemia with or without elevated platelet count. Only erythropoietin level was elevated, correlated with thrombocytosis, and decreased with iron replacement. The other cytokines remained unchanged after therapy, suggesting that they probably do not play any significant role in iron deficiency-associated reactive thrombocytosis. Recently, Bilic and Bilic reported that the amino acid sequence homology of thrombopoietin and erythropoietin may explain the thrombocytosis in children with iron deficiency anemia [103]. By contrast, two other reports suggested that the relationship between iron deficiency and reactive thrombocytosis is more complex than a mere consequence of a cross reactivity between erythropoietin and thrombopoietin [104, 105]. In addition to the increased thrombotic risk associated with high platelet count, other authors have suggested that the decrease in antioxidant defense in iron deficiency anemia may cause increased oxidant stress, which in turn may result in a tendency toward platelet aggregation [106]. Thus, the abnormal platelet count and function observed in iron deficiency anemia could act synergistically to promote thrombus formation, especially in the setting of an underlying atherosclerotic disease [107].

However, as not all cases of iron-related thrombotic events occur in patients with concomitant high platelet count [97, 98], other pathogenic mechanisms have been proposed in these last years. Thus, iron deficiency may contribute to a hyper coagulable state by affecting blood flow patterns within the vessels because of reduced deformability and increased viscosity of microcytic red blood cells [98]. Furthermore, anemic hypoxia secondary to iron deficiency could precipitate situations of increased metabolic stress (i.e., infections) in particularly vulnerable areas of the brain supplied by end arteries, such as the basal ganglia, thalamus, and hypothalamus [108]. This phenomenon could explain the association between iron-deficient anemia and reversible focal deficits and stroke found by some authors [98, 109-111].

Iron Deficiency and PICA

Pica is an irresistible craving for nonfood items that lasts at least 1 month and is developmentally inappropriate for the patient's age. Pagophagia is a specific pica for ice and was first described in association with iron deficiency in 1966. Although pica for clay can result in iron-deficiency because of impaired iron absorption, ice eating is a manifestation of existing iron deficiency. While the mechanism of this craving is unknown, the behavior is not limited to humans. An interesting study in rats demonstrated pagophagia, or a preferential eating of ice chips to meet daily water needs could be induced in animals made anemic by blood draws [112]. Pagophagia usually resolves within weeks if the iron deficiency is corrected, and a dramatic decline in ice eating can be seen within 2 weeks of starting iron therapy. The disappearance of symptoms typically occurs when fasting serum iron levels reach 70 g/100 mL or higher. Pica tends to occur in females, partly because conditions such as pregnancy and menorrhagia are common causes of iron deficiency. However, one study of adult patients with iron-deficiency anemia due to gastrointestinal blood loss still showed that females had higher rates of pica than males [113].

A study by Barton [114] et al showed that in non-pregnant adult patients with iron deficiency or depletion, lower age is a significant predictor of pica. In addition, patients with pica had lower MCV, higher RDW, and higher platelet counts than patients without pica. They identified four significant predictors of pica i.e., age and MCV (negative associations) and platelet count and RDW (positive associations).

Some reports including the above suggest that certain manifestations of iron deficiency are affected by heritable traits. *TMPRSS6* (OMIM *609862; chromosome 22q12-q13) encodes matripase-2 (trans-membrane serine protease 6). The *TMPRSS6* allele A736V (rs855791) was related to significantly lower levels of serum iron, transferring saturation, MCV, and hemoglobin in two genome-wide association studies of twins and general population subjects, respectively [115, 116]. *TMPRSS6* A736V could explain the small but significant differences observed in mean MCV and hemoglobin levels in patients with and without pica reports, although this is unproven.

A study from India [117], determined the role of trace elements in causation of pica with specific reference to zinc and iron. The plasma levels of iron (Fe), Zinc (Zn), calcium (Ca) and magnesium (Mg) and blood lead (Pb) levels were seen in 31 children with pica (Pica Group) and 60 controls matched for age, sex and nutrition. The plasma Fe level in children with pica was about 20% lower than that in controls. Plasma Zn levels in the pica group was about 45% lower than those in controls. Thus hypozincemia with low iron levels may be the possible cause of pica.

Carnitine is ingested through animal-derived foods as well as synthesized in vivo. It plays an important role in the energy metabolism of many tissues. Iron acts as a co-factor for the synthesis of carnitine. However, the importance of iron deficiency as a cause of secondary carnitine deficiency is not well established. Citak et al. [118] studied the relation of carnitine levels and PICA and showed that the mean serum carnitine concentration in the iron-deficiency group was significantly lower than that in healthy children. Based on the evidence about the effect of low iron on carnitine stores in animal studies, the authors propose that low serum carnitine levels in these children may be secondary to iron-deficiency anemia. However, further large-scale studies are needed to establish the frequency of carnitine deficiency in children with iron-deficiency anemia.

A randomized control trial by Nchito et al, studied the effect of iron and multi micronutrient supplementation on geophagy in Zambian school children. Multi micronutrients had no effect on either geophagy prevalence or earth intake. Geophagy was prevalent and associated with iron deficiency, but iron supplementation had no effects on geophageous behaviour [119].

IDA and Restless Leg Syndrome (RLS)

Restless leg syndrome is characterized by repeated aphasic involuntary muscle contractions. It is mostly reported in adult patients and largely under reported from paediatric population. Although most of the cases with RLS are idiopathic or hereditary; decreased brain iron content and metabolism can also lead to RLS. Iron deficiency states may precipitate RLS in as much as 25-30% of people. MRI studies have demonstrated decreased iron content in substantia nigra and red nucleus. Earley et al studied 16 patients of idiopathic RLS and 8 controls. They observed that patients with RLS had lower CSF ferritin and higher CSF transferrin levels than controls. Serum ferritin and transferrin levels were similar in both groups and symptoms resolved with iron therapy [121. Intravenous therapy was found to be more effective compared to oral therapy in some of the studies [120, 121]. However, it is associated with significantly increased adverse events. Although most RLS patients with low serum ferritin values are treated with oral iron therapy, no major trials on oral iron therapy are available in RLS [122].

Immune Dysfunction in Iron Deficiency

Two component systems of active immunity—humoral and cell-mediated immunity have been studied extensively, mainly in vitro, in relation to iron deficiency in both humans and animals. Little evidence exists for systematic major humoral deficiencies in iron-deficient humans, and although specific defects in cell-mediated immunity have been well described and reviewed, even in latent iron deficiency. Iron is required for normal immune function, cell differentiation and growth. Iron is also required for peroxide generating mechanisms, cytokine production and myeloperoxidase function in neutrophils. Impaired cell-mediated immunity and bactericidal function are generally noted in iron-deficient persons; however, the findings are inconsistent.

In vitro studies have reported deleterious effects of iron deficiency on cellular defences that are reversible with iron therapy. These include: a) reduced neutrophil function with decreased myeloperoxidase activity and nitro blue toluene reduction reversed by iron administration. Intracellular bactericidal activity has been reported as impaired, but not all studies give consistent results, b) depression of T-lymphocyte numbers with thymic atrophy reported in most but not all studies, c) defective T lymphocyte–induced proliferative response, d) impaired natural killer cell activity, e) impaired interleukin-2 production by lymphocytes, f) reduced production of macrophage migration inhibition factor, and g) reversible impairment of delayed cutaneous hypersensitivity, including tuberculin reactivity [123].

Certain invasive pathogens have their own powerful siderophores and iron supplementation may be deleterious in association with these infections [124]. Because of the above conflicting reports, in vivo studies in iron deficient animals and humans have been done. Animal studies revealed that effects of iron therapy are microorganism specific and that iron deficiency may be protective against intracellular pathogens. Observational studies in iron deficient humans have also revealed increased incidence of bacterial infections [125]. On the contrary, decreased malaria infection is reported in iron deficient human beings compared to controls [126, 127].

A recent review of iron intervention trials in non-malarious regions has concluded that that parenteral iron administration at birth is associated with significant risk of severe sepsis and meningitis [123]. Oral iron supplementation and food fortification was associated with significantly lower risk of respiratory infections and slight lower risk of diarrheal disease in two large studies conducted in early part of last century [128, 129]. However, four iron fortification studies conducted in late 90's failed to show any benefit or harm from iron therapy [130-133]. Contrary to this, review of iron intervention trials in malaria endemic areas has revealed that there was a significant increase in clinical malaria attack rates in 5 of 9 studies and no rate reductions; a significant increase in clinical pneumonia rates in 2 of 5 studies with no rate reductions and a significant increase in other non malarial infectious disease in 4 of 8 studies with no rate reduction [123].

To summarize, despite proven reversible functional immunological defects in vitro studies, a clinically important relationship between states of iron deficiency and susceptibility to infections remains controversial, difficult to prove and may depend on other immune factors in the community. Experimental and in vitro animal studies suggest that intracellular organisms, such as plasmodia, mycobacteria and invasive salmonellae may be enhanced by iron therapy. Besides this, no significant beneficial effect of iron supplementation has been demonstrated on immunity and infection reduction in both non-malarious and malaria endemic regions.

Conclusion

Globally iron deficiency is the commonest nutritional disorder. It is important to recognize long term consequences of iron deficiency at an individual and national level. Even though anemia is common, iron deficiency state without anemia is largely under-recognized. Mild iron deficiency without anemia also results in developmental abnormalities. Although the abnormalities may seem subtle and reversible in those children with mild iron deficiency, children with marginal iron deficiency in infancy who did not improve with iron therapy had irreversible derangement in IQ scores. Iron deficiency anemia is highly prevalent in India (reported 55.7% to 85.1% in different states in NFHS-3)[134] and much larger population having iron deficiency without anemia. It is estimated that the effect of ID on cognitive losses during childhood results in an estimated 2.5% loss of earnings during adulthood. Given the high proportion of the population with ID or anemia in most developing countries, interventions to improve the iron status of young children should be given high priority. New insights into the biology of early development and the role of iron in neurodevelopment will eventually allow public health professionals to better design and target these interventions. Hence, it is critical that measures are undertaken to detect and treat ID and IDA as early as possible.

References

[1] World Health Organisation. *Worldwide Prevalence of Anaemia 1993–2005: WHO Global Database on Anaemia*. de Benoist B, McLean E, Egli I, Cogswell M, eds. Geneva, Switzerland: WHO Press; 2008.

[2] McLean E, Egli I, de Benoist B, Wojdyla D, Cogswell M. Worldwide prevalence of anemia in pre-school aged children, pregnant women and non-pregnant women of reproductive age. In: Kraemer K, Zimmermann MB, eds. *Nutritional Anemia*. Basel, Switzerland: Sight and Life Press; 2007:1–12.

[3] Lozoff B, Jimenez E, Smith JB. Double burden of iron deficiency in infancy and low socioeconomic status: a longitudinal analysis of cognitive test scores to age 19 years. *Arch Pediatr Adolesc Med*. 2006; 160(11):1108–1113.

[4] Bruner AB, Joffe A, Duggan AK, Casella JF, Brandt J. Randomized study of cognitive effects of iron supplementation in nonanemic iron-deficient adolescent girls. *Lancet*, 1996;348(9033):992–996.

[5] Oppenheimer SJ. Iron and its relation to immunity and infectious disease. *J Nutr*. 2001;131:S616–633.

[6] Haas JD, Brownlie IV. Iron deficiency and reduced work capacity: a critical review of the research to determine a causal relationship. *J Nutr*. 2001;13: S676–690.

[7] Sachdev HPS, Gera T, Nestel P. Effect of iron supplementation on physical growth in children: systematic review of randomised controlled trials. Public *Health Nutr.* 2006;9:904– 920.

[8] Lozoff B, Jimenez E, Hagen J, Mollen E, Wolf AW. Poorer behavioral and developmental outcome more than 10 years after treatment for iron deficiency in infancy. *Pediatrics*, 2000;105:E51.

[9] Lozoff B, Beard J, Connor J, Barbara F, Georgieff M, Schallert T. Long-lasting neural and behavioral effects of iron deficiency in infancy. *Nutr Rev*. 2006;64:S34–43.

[10] Stoltzfus RJ, Kvalsvig JD, Chwaya HM, et al. Effects of iron supplementation and anthelmintic treatment on motor and language development of preschool children in Zanzibar: double blind, placebo controlled study. *BMJ*. 2001;323:1389– 1393.

[11] Beard J. Recent evidence from human and animal studies regarding iron status and infant development. *J. Nutr*. 2007;137:S524–530.

[12] Black RE, Allen LH, Bhutta ZA, et al. Maternal and child undernutrition: global and regional exposures and health consequences. *Lancet*, 2008; 371:243–260.

[13] Copenhagen Business School. Global Crises, Global Solutions: Costs and Benefits. Cambridge: Cambridge University Press; 2009.

[14] Horton S, Alderman H. The economics of addressing nutritional anemia. In: Kraemer K, Zimmermann MB, eds. Nutritional Anemia. Zurich: Sight and Life Press; 2007: 19–35.

[15] World Health Organization. Iron Deficiency Anemia: Assessment, Prevention, and Control— A Guide for Program Managers. Geneva, Switzerland: World Health Organization; 2001. WHO/NHD/01.3.

[16] Centers for Disease Control and Prevention, National Center for Health Statistics. National Health and Nutrition Examination Survey. Available at: www.cdc.gov/ nchs/nhanes.htm.

[17] Cusick SE, Mei Z, Freedman DS, et al. Unexplained decline in the prevalence of anemia among US children and women between 1988 –1994 and 1999 –2002. *Am J Clin Nutr*. 2008;88:1611–1617.

[18] Pollycove M: Iron metabolism and kinetics. *Semin Hematol*. 1966;3:235.

[19] Ohira Y, Cartier LJ, Chen M, Holloszy JO: Induction of an increase in mitochondrial matrix enzymes in muscle of iron-deficient rats. *Am J Physiol*. 1987;253:C639.

[20] Finch CA, Gollnick PD, Hlastala MP, et al: Lactic acidosis as a result of iron deficiency. *J Clin Invest*. 1979;64:129.

[21] MacDonald VW, Charache S, Hathaway PJ: Iron deficiency anemia: Mitochondrial alpha-glycerophosphate dehydrogenase in guinea pig skeletal muscle. *J Lab Clin Med*. 1985;105:11.

[22] Mackler B, Person R, Grace R: Iron deficiency in the rat: Effects on energy metabolism in brown adipose tissue. Pediatr Res 1985;19:989.

[23] Walter PB, Knutson MD, Paler-Martinez A, et al: Iron deficiency and iron excess damage mitochondria and mitochondrial DNA in rats. *Proc Natl Acad Sci USA*. 2002;99:2264.

[24] Harlan WR, Williams RS: Activity-induced adaptations in skeletal muscles of iron-deficient rabbits. *J Appl Physiol*. 1988;65:782.

[25] Evans TC, Mackler B: Effect of iron deficiency on energy conservation in rat liver and skeletal muscle submitochondrial particles. *Biochem Med.* 1985;34:93.

[26] Thompson CH, Green YS, Ledingham JG, et al: The effect of iron deficiency on skeletal muscle metabolism of the rat. *Acta Physiol Scand.* 1993;147:85.

[27] Thompson CH, Kemp GJ, Taylor DJ, et al: No evidence of mitochondrial abnormality in skeletal muscle of patients with iron-deficient anaemia. *J Intern Med.* 1993;234:149.

[28] Hinton PS, Sinclair LM: Iron supplementation maintains ventilatory threshold and improves energetic efficiency in iron-deficient nonanemic athletes. *Eur J Clin Nutr.* 2007;61:30.

[29] Brownlie T, Utermohlen V, Hinton PS, Haas JD: Tissue iron deficiency without anemia impairs adaptation in endurance capacity after aerobic training in previously untrained women. *Am J Clin Nutr.* 2004;79:437.

[30] Hinton PS, Giordano C, Brownlie T, Haas JD: Iron supplementation improves endurance after training in iron-depleted, nonanemic women. *J Appl Physiol.* 2000;88:1103.

[31] Youdim MB, Ben Shachar D: Minimal brain damage induced by early iron deficiency: Modified dopaminergic neurotransmission. *Isr J Med Sci.* 1987;23:19.

[32] Fischbach MA, Lin H, Liu DR, Walsh CT: How pathogenic bacteria evade mammalian sabotage in the battle for iron. *Nat Chem Biol.* 2006;2:132.

[33] Black MM, Lozoff B. Nutrition and child development. In: Haith MM, Benson JB, eds. Encyclopedia of Infant and Child Development. Oxford, UK: Elsevier Inc.; 2008: 449–459.

[34] Lozoff B, Georgieff MK. Iron deficiency and brain development. *Semin Pediatr Neurol.* 2006;13:158–165.

[35] Grantham-McGregor S, Ani C. A review of studies on the effect of iron deficiency on cognitive development in children. *J Nutr.* 2001;131:S649–666.

[36] Lozoff B, Jimenez E, Smith JB. Double burden of iron deficiency in infancy and low socioeconomic status: a longitudinal analysis of cognitive test scores to age 19 years. *Arch Pediatr Adolesc Med.* 2006;160:1108–1113.

[37] Beard J. Iron deficiency alters brain development and functioning. *J Nutr.* 2003;133:S1468–S1472.

[38] Taylor EM, Crowe A, Morgan EH. Transferrin and iron uptake by the brain: effects of altered iron status. *J Neurochem.* 1991;57:1584–1592.

[39] Crowe A, Morgan EH. Iron and transferrin uptake by brain and cerebrospinal fluid in the rat. *Brain Res.* 1992;592:8–16.

[40] Han J, Day JR, Connor JR, Beard JL. Gene expression of transferrin and transferrin receptor in brains of control vs. irondeficient rats. *Nutr Neurosci.* 2003;6:1–10.

[41] Rao R, Tkac I, Townsend EL, Gruetter R, Georgieff MK. Perinatal iron deficiency alters the neurochemical profile of the developing rat hippocampus. *J Nutr.* 2003;133:3215–3221.

[42] Beard JL. Why iron deficiency is important in infant development. *J Nutr.* 2008;138:2534–2536.

[43] Beard JL,Wiesinger JA, Connor JR. Pre- and postweaning iron deficiency alters myelination in Sprague-Dawley rats. *Dev Neurosci.* 2003;25:308–315.

[44] Bianco LE, Wiesinger J, Earley CJ, Jones BC, Beard JL. Iron deficiency alters dopamine uptake and response to L-DOPA injection in Sprague-Dawley rats. *J Neurochem*. 2008;106: 205–215.

[45] Burhans MS, Dailey C, Beard Z, et al. Iron deficiency: differential effects on monoamine transporters. *Nutr Neurosci*. 2005;8:31–38.

[46] Burhans MS, Dailey C, Wiesinger J, Murray-Kolb LE, Jones BC, Beard JL. Iron deficiency affects acoustic startle response and latency, but not prepulse inhibition in young adult rats. *Physiol Behav*. 2006;87:917–924.

[47] Dwork AJ, Lawler G, Zybert PA, et al. An autoradiographic study of the uptake and distribution of iron by the brain of the young rat. *Brain Res*. 1990;518:31–39.

[48] Aoki S, Okada Y, Nishimura K, et al. Normal deposition of brain iron in childhood and adolescence: MR imaging at 1.5 T. *Radiology*. 1989;172:381–385.

[49] Beard JL, Connor JD, Jones BC. Brain iron: location and function. *Prog Food Nutr Sci*. 1993;17:183–221.

[50] Beard JL, Unger EL, Bianco LE, Paul T, Rundle SE, Jones BC. Early postnatal iron repletion overcomes lasting effects of gestational iron deficiency in rats. *J Nutr*. 2007;137:1176– 1182.

[51] Felt BT, Lozoff B. Brain iron and behavior of rats are not normalized by treatment of iron deficiency anemia during early development. *J Nutr*. 1996;126:693–701.

[52] Lozoff B. Iron deficiency and child development. *Food Nutr Bull*. 2007;28:S560–571.

[53] Sachdev HPS, Gera T, Nestel P. Effect of iron supplementation on mental and motor development in children: systematic review of randomised controlled trials. *Public Health Nutr*. 2005;8:117–132.

[54] Lynn R, Harland EP. A positive effect of iron supplementation on the IQs of iron deficient children. *Pers Individ Dif*. 1998;24:883–885.

[55] Seshadri S, Gopaldas T. Impact of iron supplementation on cognitive functions in preschool and school-aged children – the Indian experience. *Am J Clin Nutr*. 1989;50:675–686.

[56] Roncagliolo M, Garrido M, Walter T, Peirano P, Lozoff B. Evidence of altered central nervous system development in infants with iron deficiency anemia at 6 mo: delayed maturation of auditory brainstem responses. *Am J Clin Nutr*. 1998;68:683–690.

[57] Burden MJ, Westerlund AJ, Armony-Sivan R, et al. An eventrelated potential study of attention and recognition memory in infants with iron-deficiency anemia. *Pediatrics*, 2007; 120:e336–e345.

[58] Lozoff B, Clark KM, Jing Y, Armony-Sivan R, Angelilli ML, Jacobson SW. Dose-response relationships between iron deficiency with or without anemia and infant socialemotional behavior. *J Pediatr*. 2008;152:696–702.

[59] Freeman JM. Febrile seizures: a consensus of their significance, evaluation, and treatment. *Pediatrics*, 1980; 66:1009-1012.

[60] Hauser WA. The prevalence and incidence of convulsive disorders in children. *Epilepsia*. 1994;35:S1-S6.

[61] Shinnar S, Glauser TA. Febrile seizures. J Child Neurol 2002;17:S44-S52.

[62] Camfield P, Camfield C, Gordon K. Antecedents and Risk Factors for Febrile Seizures. San Diego, CA: Academic Press; 2002.

[63] Beard JL. Iron biology in immune function, muscle metabolism and neuronal functioning. *J Nutr*. 2001;131: 568S-579S.

[64] Ghosh K. Non haematological effects of iron deficiency: a perspective. *Indian J Med Sci.* 2006;60:30-37.

[65] Yager JY, Hartfield DS. Neurologic manifestations of iron deficiency in childhood. *Pediatr Neurol.* 2002;27: 85-92.

[66] Kobrinsky NL, Yager JY, Cheang MS, et al. Does iron deficiency raise the seizure threshold? *J Child Neurol.* 1995;10:105-109.

[67] Pisacane A, Sansone R, Impagliazzo N, et al. Iron deficiency anaemia and febrile convulsions: case-control study in children under 2 years. *BMJ.* 1996;313:343.

[68] Daoud AS, Batieha A, Abu-Ekteish F, et al. Iron status: a possible risk factor for the first febrile seizure. *Epilepsia.* 2002;43:740-743.

[69] Naveed-ur R, Billoo AG. Association between iron deficiency anemia and febrile seizures. *J Coll Physicians Surg Pak.* 2005;15:338-340.

[70] Hartfield DS, Tan J, Yager JY, Rosychuk RJ, Spady D, Haines C, Craig WR. The association between iron deficiency and febrile seizures in childhood. *Clin Pediatr (Phila).* 2009;48(4):420-6.

[71] Millichap JG, Millichap JJ. Role of viral infections in the etiology of febrile seizures. *Pediatr Neurol.* 2006;35:165-172.

[72] Nakayama J, Arinami T. Molecular genetics of febrile seizures. *Epilepsy Res.* 2006;70:S190-S198.

[73] Colina KF, Abelson HT. Resolution of breath-holding spells with treatment of concomitant anemia. *J Pediatr.* 1995;**126**:395–397.

[74] Daoud AS, Batieha A, Al-sheyyab M, Abuekteish F, Hijazi S. Effectiveness of iron therapy on breath-holding spells. *J Pediatr.* 1997;**130:**547–550.

[75] Holowach J, Thurston DL. Breath-holding spells and anemia. *N Engl J Med.* 1963; **268**:21–23.

[76] Samuels MP, Talber DG, Southall DP. Cyanotic breathholding and sudden death. *Archives of Disease in Childhood*, 1991;66:257–8.

[77] Poets CF, Samuels MP,Wardrop CAJ, Picton-Jones E, Southall DP. Reduced haemoglobin levels in infants presenting with apparent life treating events: a retrospective investigation. *Acta Pediatrica*, 1992; 81:319–21.

[78] Mocan MC, Mocan H, Aslan Y, Erduran E. Iron therapy in breathholding spells and cerebral erythropoetin [letter]. *Journal of Pediatrics*, 1998;133:583–4.

[79] Oski FA, Honig AS. The effects on the developmental scores of iron-deficient infants. *Journal of Pediatrics*, 1978;92:21–5.

[80] Masuda S, Okano M, Yamagishi K, Nagao M, Ueda M, Sasaki R. A novel site of erythropoietin production: oxygen-dependent production in cultured rat astrocytes. *Journal of Biological Chemistry*, 1994;269:19488–93.

[81] Bhatia MS, Singhal PK, Dhar NK, Nigam VR, Malik SC, Mullick K. Breath holding spells: An analysis of 50 cases. *Indian Pediatr.* 1990; **27:**1073–1079.

[82] Bruggers CS, Ware R, Altman AJ, Rourk MH, Vedanarayanan V, Chaffee S. Reversible focal neurologic deficits in severe iron deficiency anemia. *J Pediatr.* 1990;**117**:430–432.

[83] Forster HS. Optic disc edema due to iron deficiency. *Conn Med.* 1985;**49**:290–292.

[84] Parag KB, Omar MAK. Benign intracranial hypertension associated with iron deficiency anaemia. *S Afr Med J.* 1983;**63**:981–982.

[85] Pless M, Lipton SA. Iron deficiency in children. *N Engl J Med.* 1993;**329:**1741.

[86] Stoebner R, Kiser R, Alperin JB. Iron deficiency anemia and papilledema: Rapid resolution with oral iron therapy. *Am J Dig Dis*;190;**15**:919–922.

[87] Trujillo MH, Desenne JJ, Benaim Pinto H. Reversible papilledema in iron deficiency anemia: Two cases with normal spinal fluid pressure. *Ann Ophthalmol.* 1972**; 4:** 378–380.

[88] Tugal O, Jacobson R, Berezin S. Recurrent benign intracranial hypertension due to iron deficiency anemia: Case report and review of the literature. *Am J Pediatr Hematol Oncol.* 1994;**16**:266–270.

[89] Clark A. Observations on the anaemia or chlorosis of girls, occurring more commonly between the advent of menstruation and the consummation of womanhood. Lancet 1887;ii:1003–1005.

[90] Osler W. The principles and practice of medicine. 4th ed., Appelton and Co., New York 1901;pp. 792–795.

[91] Von Dusch T (1861) On thrombosis of the cerebral sinuses. The New Sydenham Society, London.

[92] Vaitl J (1895) Zur Aetiologie und Pathogenese der autochthonen Sinusthrombose. Thesis University of Munich.

[93] Leichtenstern O. Ueber Venenthrombose bei Chlorose. Mu¨nchner Med Wochenschr 1899;48:1603–1606.

[94] Dan K. Thrombocytosis in iron deficiency anemia. *Intern Med.* 2005;44:1025–1026.

[95] Dickeroff R, von Ruecker A. Thrombozytose im Kindesalter. Differential diagnose und klinische Bedeutung. Paediatrische Praxis 1991;41:25–28 .

[96] Nagai T, Komatsu N, Sakata Y, Miura Y, Ozawa K. Iron deficiency anemia with marked thrombocytosis complicated by central retinal vein occlusion. *Intern Med.* 2005; 44:1090–1092

[97] Kinoshita Y, Taniura S, Shishido H, Nojima T, Kamitani H, Watanebe T. Cerebral venous sinus thrombosis associated with iron deficiency: two case reports. *Neurol Med Chir.* (Tokyo) 2006;46:589–593

[98] Hartfield DS, Lowry NJ, Keene DL, Yager JY. Iron deficiency: a cause of stroke in infants and children. *Pediatr Neurol.* 1997;16:50–53.

[99] Stolz E, Valdueza JM, Grebe M, Schlachetzki F, Schmitt E, Madlener K, Rahimi A, Kempkes-Matthes B, Blaes F, Gerriets T, Kaps M. Anemia as a risk factor for cerebral venous thrombosis? An old hypothesis revisited: results of a prospective study. *J Neurol.* 2007;254:729–734

[100] Karpatkin S, Garg S, Freedman M. Role of iron as a regulator of thrombopoiesis. *Am J Med.* 1974;57:521–525

[101] Beguin Y. Erythropoietin and platelet production. *Haematologica*, 1999;84:541–547

[102] Akan H, Guven N, Aydogdu I, Arat M, Beksac M, Dalva K. Thrombopoietic cytokines in patients with iron deficiency anemia with or without thrombocytosis. *Acta Haematol.* 2000;103:152–156.

[103] Bilic E, Bilic E. Amino acid sequence homology of thrombopoietin and erythropoietin may explain thrombocytosis in children with iron deficiency anemia. *J Pediatr Hematol Oncol.* 2003;25:675–676.

[104] Racke F. EPO and TPO sequences do not explain thrombocytosis in iron deficiency anemia. *J Pediatr Hematol Oncol.* 2003;25:919.

[105] Geddis AE, Kaushansky K. Cross-reactivity between erythropoietin and thrombopoietin at the level of Mpl does not account for the thrombocytosis seen in iron deficiency. *J Pediatr Hematol Oncol*. 2003;25:919–920.

[106] Tekin D, Yavuzer S, Tekin M, Akar N, Cin S. Possible effects of antioxidant status on increased platelet aggregation in childhood iron-deficiency anemia. *Pediatr Int*. 2001;43:74–77

[107] Akins PT, Glenn S, Nemeth PM, Derdeyn CP. Carotid artery thrombus associated with severe iron-deficiency anemia and thrombocytosis. *Stroke*, 1996; 27:1002–1005

[108] Balci K, Utku U, Asil T, Buyukkoyuncu N. Deep cerebral vein thrombosis associated with iron deficiency anaemia in adults. *J Clin Neurosci*. 2007;14:181–184.

[109] Young RS, Rannels DE, Hilmo A, Gerson JM, Goodrich D. Severe anemia in childhood presenting as transient ischemic attacks. *Stroke*, 1983;14:622–623

[110] Hart RG, Kanter MG. Hematologic disorders and ischemic stroke. A selective review. *Stroke*, 1990;21:1111–1121

[111] Gillum RF, Sempos CT, Makuc DM, Looker AC, Chien CY, Ingram DD. Serum transferrin saturation, stroke incidence, and mortality in women and men. The NHANES I Epidemiologic Followup Study. National Health and Nutrition Examination Survey. *Am J Epidemiol*. 1996;144:59–68

[112] Woods SC, Weisinger RS. Pagophagia in the albino rat. Science. 1970;169:1334-1336.

[113] Rector, WG Jr. Pica: its frequency and significance in patients with iron-deficiency anemia due to chronic gastrointestinal blood loss. *J Gen Intern Med*. 1989; 4:512-513.

[114] Barton JC, Barton JC, Bertoli LF. Pica associated with iron deficiency or depletion: clinical and laboratory correlates in 262 non-pregnant adult outpatients. *BMC Blood Disord*. 2010 22;10:9.

[115] Chambers JC, Zhang W, Li Y, Sehmi J, Wass MN, Zabaneh D, Hoggart C, Bayele H, McCarthy MI, Peltonen L. et al. Genome-wide association study identifies variants in *TMPRSS6* associated with hemoglobin levels. *Nat Genet*. 2009;**41**:1170–1172.

[116] Mizuno S, Mihara T, Miyaoka T, Inagaki T, Horiguchi J. CSF iron, ferritin and transferrin levels in restless legs syndrome. *J Sleep Res*. 2005;**14**:43–47.

[117] Singhi S, Ravishanker R, Singhi P, Nath R. Low plasma zinc and iron in pica. Indian *J Pediatr*. 2003;70(2):139-43.

[118] Citak EC, Citak FE, Kurekci AE. Serum carnitine levels in children with iron-deficiency anemia with or without pica. *Pediatr Hematol Oncol*. 2006;23(5):381- 5.

[119] Nchito M, Geissler PW, Mubila L, Friis H, Olsen A. The effect of iron and multi-micronutrient supplementation on Ascaris lumbricoides reinfection among Zambian schoolchildren. *Trans R Soc Trop Med Hyg*. 2009;103(3):229-36.

[120] Earley CJ, Heckler D, Allen RP. The treatment of restless legs syndrome with intravenous iron dextran. *Sleep Med*. 2004; 5:231–5.

[121] Sloand JA, Shelly MA, Feigin A, et al. A doubleblind, placebo-controlled trial of intravenous iron dextran therapy in patients with ESRD and restless legs syndrome. *Am J Kidney Dis*. 2004; 43:663–70.

[122] Trenkwalder C, Hogl B,Winkelmann J. Recent advances in diagnosis, genetics and treatment of Restless leg Syndrome. *J Neurol*. 2009; 256:539-53.

[123] Oppenheimer SJ. Iron and its relation to immunity and infectious disease. *J Nutr*. 2001; 131:616S-635S.

[124] Oppenheimer SJ, Hendrickse RG. The clinical effects of iron deficiency and iron supplementation. *Nutr Abstr Rev*. 1983; 53: 585–98.

[125] Harju E. Empty iron stores as a significant risk factor in abdominal surgery. *J Parent Enteral Nutr*. 1988; 12:282–5.

[126] Oppenheimer S J, Gibson FD, Macfarlane SBJ, et al. Iron supplementation increases prevalence and effects of malaria. Report on clinical studies in Papua New Guinea. *Trans R Soc Trop Med Hyg*. 1986; 80:603–12.

[127] Oppenheimer SJ, Macfarlane SBJ, Moody JB, et al. Effect of iron prophylaxis on morbidity due to infectious disease. Report on clinical studies in Papua New Guinea. *Trans R Soc Trop Med Hyg*. 1986; 80:596–602.

[128] MacKay H M. Anaemia in infancy; its prevalence and prevention. *Arch Dis Child*. 1928; 3:117–47.

[129] Andelman MB, Sered BR. Utilization of dietary iron by term infants. A study of 1,048 infants from a low socioeconomic population. *Am. J. Dis Child*. 1966; 111: 45–55.

[130] Power HM, Heese HD, Beatty DW, et al. Iron fortification of infant formula: the effect on iron status and immune function. *Ann. Trop Paediatr*. 1991; 11:57–66.

[131] Hemminki E, Nemet K, Horvath M, et al. Impact of iron fortification of milk formulas on infant's growth and health. *Nutr. Res*. 1995; 15:491–503.

[132] Javaid N, Haschke F, Pietschnig B, et al. Interactions between infections, malnutrition and iron nutritional status in Pakistani infants. *Acta Paediatr Scand Suppl*. 1991; 80:141–50.

[133] Mitra AK, Akramuzzaman SM, Fuchs GJ, et al. Long-term oral supplementation with iron is not harmful for young children in a poor community of Bangladesh. *J Nutr*. 1997; 127:1451–5.

[134] National Family Health Survey-3, 2005-2006. International Institute of Population Sciences, Mumbai 2005.

In: Iron Deficiency and Its Complications
Editor: Yildiz Dincer
ISBN 978-1-61324-854-6

Chapter 3

Iron Metabolism and Consequences of Iron Deficiency

Yildiz Dincer
Istanbul University Cerrahpasa Medical Faculty,
Department of Biochemistry, Istanbul, Turkey

ABSTRACT

Iron is a trace element, as it is required for erythropoiesis, oxidative metabolism, cellular immune response, and some of hormonal functions and enzymatic activity. Iron is distributed in the body in various compartments including hemoglobin, myoglobin, tissue iron and a labile pool. Transport of iron from one organ to another is accomplished by transferrin. The major pathway of iron metabolism is a closed cycle in which iron passes from plasma transferrin to red blood cell precursors in the bone marrow, where it is used in hemoglobin synthesis; these cells then enter the circulation in the form of mature red blood cells, where they remain nearly 120 days before they are degredated; the iron is released from hemoglobin and returns to plasma transferrin, thus completing one cycle and starting a new one. From this iron cycle, small quantities of iron are diverted for use in other iron compartments. Iron deficiency is one of the most prevalent disorder of humans. Increased iron requirements, limited external supply, and increased blood loss may lead to iron deficiency. Its causes can consist of many overlapping factor. In the initial phase of iron depletion, iron stores maintain normal levels of hemoglobin and other iron compounds. With exhaustion of iron store hypochromic and microcytic anemia becomes manifest. Iron deficiency anemia has been associated with growth retardation and lower neuronal development in infants and has long-lasting effects on mental and motor functions in spite of normalization of hematological status and growth. Adults with iron deficiency anemia have reduced attention spans and work capacity. Numerious cellular enzymes and coenzymes require iron, either as an integral part of their structure or as a cofactor. Therefore, iron is essential in various biochemical pathways required for neuronal function. Iron is required for thyroid hormon synthesis. The prevalance of iron deficiency among children living in areas of endemic goiter is high. Impaired muscle performance has been determined in iron deficiency. Chronic iron deficiency has been reported not only as a primary cause, but also as a facilitator of heart failure. Deficits in iron functional compartments have suppressive effects on the immune system. Taken together, it is clear that iron has a pivotal role in the maintenance of normal metabolic funtion and iron deficiency leads serious consequences. This chapther will review what is currently known about pathological consequences of iron deficiency and what are the mechanisms underlying these pathologies.

INTRODUCTION

Iron is an essential micronutrient and is vital for all cells. It is requied at many points in the metabolism. Heme is an iron-porphyrin complex. It is the prosthetic group of many important proteins such as hemoglobin, myoglobin, cytochromes, peroxidases, catalase. Iron also participates in a variety of reactions as non-heme iron. Hemoglobin and myoglobin have a central role in oxygen transport and storage, respectively. As a transition metal ion, iron is able to switch between multiple oxidation states. This makes it an important co-factor in electron transfer and redox reactions needed for synthesis of metabolically important compounds and for degradation and detoxification of waste products and environmental toxins [1].

ABSORBTION OF IRON

Total body iron of a 70-kg adult is about 4-4,5 g. The dietary requirement of iron depends on the amount of the iron lost from the body, and variations in physiological state such as growth, pregnancy and onset of menses. Absorption of dietary iron is tightly regulated, and is solely balanced with losses. Very little iron is lost from the body, and it is mainly from loss of cells in the gastrointestinal tract and to a lesser extent from the skin and in the urine. The iron excreted in women averages more than that in men because of menstrual blood loss. As a transition metal ion, iron can generate free radicals via Fenton reaction; therefore, iron overload and abnormal metabolism of iron can lead to several chronic pathogenesis. Free radical-mediated oxidative stress is one of the major causative factors for diabetes and diabetic complications. Thus, both iron deficiency and iron excess can have adverse effects on a variety of cell, tissue and organ functions. Iron blance is maintained by control of absorbtion. In iron deficiency the percentage of iron absorbed from the diet can increase to 20 to 30%. Iron in food exist mainly in the ferric (Fe^{3+}) state, complexed to proteins, amino acids, organic acids or heme. The major providers of the iron are meat and legume family. Iron is absorbed mainly in the duodenum, to a smaller extent also in the upper jejunum. It is absorbed both in ionized form and as heme iron. Heme iron is absorbed more efficiently than ionized iron. Ionized iron exist in foods mainly in the ferric state can be absorbed in the ferrous (Fe^{2+}) state and has to be reduced prior to transport. Reduction of dieatry ferric iron to ferrous iron is accomplished by the ferric reductase (Dcytb) located on the luminal intestinal membrane. Ascorbic acid, as a reducing substance, contributes to reduction of ferric iron to ferrous form [1]. Reduced iron (Fe^{2+}) is than transported by divalent metal transporter 1 (DMT1), the intestinal iron importer. DMT1 also transports other metal ions such as zinc, copper and cobalt by a proton coupled mechanism [2]. Gastric acid potentiates iron absorption by helping in formation of soluble and absorbable ferrous chelats. In achlorhydria iron absorbtion is subnormal. Iron absorbtion is also inhibited by carbonates, phosphates, phytates, tannins, phenolic compounds (coffee , tea), tetracyclines and gastric anti-acid agents and antisecretory drugs [3]. Absorbtion of heme iron is not affected by these agents because heme is absorbed as intact from foods. Heme binds to a heme receptor on the luminal surface of the enterocytes and is taken up into the intestinal cell by endocytosis. The iron is cleaved from the porphyrine ring by hemoxygenase and is released to cytoplasm, so that it is available for the production of iron containing enzymes and for delivery to the body [4].

Once inside the intestinal epithelial cell, the iron may either remains in the cell for use or storage or transported into the circulation. A renewed valency change is required before iron can be transported. Ferrous iron once exported across the basal membrane by ferroportin 1 is then oxidized by a multi-copper oxidase protein called hephaestin, a copper-containing transmembrane ferroxidase on the basolateral membrane of enterocytes [5]. Ferroportin 1 is also the putative iron exporter in macrophages and hepatocytes. The distribution of the iron entering the portal blood from the mucosal cell takes play by binding to a specific transport protein, transferrin. This protein is synthesized in the liver. Each molecule of apotransferrin can bind two atoms of iron in the ferric state . Under physiological conditions approximately 30%-40% of the binding sites are occupied by iron. Transferrin levels correlate inversely with the amount of body iron stores. Transferrin binds to transferrin receptors on the cell membrane of erythroid precursors, reticulocytes and most body cells. Transferrin-bound iron is the major iron source for most tissues. The transferin-receptor complex is rapidly internalized, iron is released, and apotransferrin returns to the circulation and binds more iron. The transferrin receptors density depends on the iron requirement of the cell. The concentration of soluble transferrin receptors in plasma is increased in absolute iron deficiency [6].

Iron is stored in the cytosolic iron storage molecule, ferritin. Ferritin is a water-soluble complex of ferric salt and a protein, apoferritin. Apoferritin forms a shell around a cyrstalline core of predominatelly ferric oxyhydroxide. Ferritin is present throughout the reticuloendothelial system and in the parenchyma of many organs such as liver and muscle as well in body fluids. Although ferritin is an intracellular iron storage protein, small amounts of ferritin are secreted into the circulation. Plasma ferritin concentration correlates well with the iron stores. 1 ng/mL serum ferritin corresponds to approximately 8 mg of stored iron. Another substance mediates to iron storage is hemosiderin. Hemosiderin is water-insoluble iron complex. It consists mostly of aggregates of ferric oxyhydroxide core cyristalls and is thought to be a breakdown product of ferritin. Hemosiderin is present particularly in the reticuloendothelial cells of the bone marrow, liver and spleen.

The absorption of iron is dependent on the body's iron stores, hypoxia and rate of erythropoiesis. Two models have been proposed to explain the regulation of iron absorbtion: the crypt programming model and the hepcidin model [3]

1. The Crypt Programming Model

The intracellular iron level of the crypt cells of the duodenum corresponds to the body's iron stores, which in turn determines the amount of iron absorbed from the intestine, as these crypt cells migrate upwards to become absorptive cells at the brush border. The intracellular iron concentration controls the interaction of cytosolic iron regulatory proteins (IRP) 1 and 2 with iron regulatory elements (IRE). IRE act as iron sensors in mammalian cells and regulate translation of mRNA of transferin receptor 1, DMT-1, ferroportin1, and ferritin. In the absence of iron, IRP1 binds to IRE of TfR1, DMT-1, and ferroportin 1 mRNA, the transcription is stimulated and these proteins are synthesized. Thus, absorbtion of dietary iron increases. When IRP bind to IRE of ferritin mRNA, translation of the transcript is blocked and synthesis of ferritin is suppressed. Therefore, ferritin levels are regulated reciprocally: it is increased in iron-replete states and is decreased in iron deficiency.

2. The Hepcidin Model

Hepcidine is a iron-regulatory hormone. It is synthesized by the liver in response to an increase in transferrin saturation. It plays a major role in regulating iron homeostasis [7]. Once secreted into the circulation, hepcidin binds ferroportin on enterocytes, macrophages and hepatic cells, which triggers its internalization and lysosomal degradation. Thus, hepcidine functions to decrease serum iron levels by blocking iron absorption from the intestine, iron recycling from macrophages, and mobilization of stored iron from liver hepatocytes [8]. Under phsiological conditions hepcidin production increases in response to iron loading and decreases in iron deficiency. Such regulation of hepcidin expression serves to modulate iron absorption to meet body iron demand. Hepcidin expression is also regulated by erythroid factors, hypoxia, and inflammation, regardless of body iron levels [9]. In hepcidin excess, ferroportin is inhibited, gastrointestinal iron absorption and iron releasing from macrophages and hepatocytes are diminished. Consequently, serum iron is decreased resulting in decreased delivery of iron to the bone marrow and therefore iron deficiency anemia develops, even in the presence of adequate total iron stores. This situation is called as functional iron deficiency.

Functions of Iron

Iron takes part in oxygen transport, oxygen storage, electron transport and some enzymatic reactions in the form of either heme or inorganic iron. Approximately 65–75% of the total body iron is found in the hemoglobin of red blood cells. The liver stores 10–20% in the form of ferritin, which can be mobilized easily when needed. About 3–4% of the body's iron is in myoglobin in striated muscle. The rest is distributed in other tissues and used in other metabolic reactions. Iron containing biomolecules and their funtions are shown in the Table 1.

Heme-Iron

Hemoglobin and Myoglobin

The central role of hemoglobin and myoglobin in oxygen transport and storage is well known. Both hemoglobin and myoglobin contain Fe^{2+}-porphyrin complex known as heme group. Oxygen binding occurs at the heme iron. Hemoglobin is predominant protein in red blood cells and is responsible for transporting oxygen, carbon dioxide, and protons between the lungs and tissues. Proton transport from tissues to lungs contributes to acide-base balance in the body [1]. Myoglobin is a heme protein found in high concentrations in red muscle, particularly in cardiac muscle. It is responsible for oxygen storage in muscles and oxygen releasing in the case of very low oxygen pressure in muscles [1].

Table 1. Iron containing biomolecules and their functions

Biomolecule	Function
Heme-iron	
Hemoglobin	Oxygen transporting
Myoglobin	Oxygen storing in the muscles
Cytochromes	Mitochondrial ATP production
	Detoxification
	Synthesis of cholesterol and cholesterol derived biomolecules (bile acids, vitamin D, estrogens, androgens, mineralocorticoids, glucocorticoids)
Cytochrome oxidase	ATP production
Glutathione peroxidase	Antioxidant defence
Catalase	Antioxidant defence
Thyroperoxidase	Thyroid hormone synthesis
NADPH oxidase	Immune defence
Myeloperoxidase	Immune defence
Acyl coenzyme A desaturases	Polyunsaturated fatty acid synthesis
Guanylyl Cyclase	NO-mediated vasodilation
Methemoglobin reductase	Conversion of methemoglobin to hemoglobin
Tyrptophan pyrrolase	Tyrptophan catabolism-nicotinic acid synthesis
Nitric oxide synthase	NO production
Non-heme-iron	
Fe-S clusters	Mitochondrial ATP production
Aconitase	Citric acid cycle
Ribonucleotide reductase	DNA synthesis
NADH dehydrogenase	Citric acid cycle
Succinate dehydrogenase	Citric acid cycle

Cytochromes

The cytochromes are iron-containing hemoproteins in which the iron atom oscillates between Fe^{2+} and Fe^{3+} states during the oxido-reduction reactions. Cytochromes are differentiated on the basis of their apoprotein structure, heme structure, and optical absorbtion of reduced state in the visible spectrum [10]. The mitochondrial electron transfer chain contains at least six different cytochrome. Cytochromes also participate various metabolic reactions as an integral part of cellular enzymes and coenzymes. In this way, they contribute to antioxidant defence, thyroid hormone biosynthesis, immune defence, metabolism of various endogenous biomolecules, detoxification of xenobiotics, fatty acid biosynthesis and prostaglandin biosynthesis [11].

Nicotinamide Adenine Dinucleotide (NADH)-Cytochrome B5 Reductase (Methemoglobin Reductase)

Methemoglobin is the derivative of hemoglobin in which the iron of the heme group is oxidized to the Fe^{3+} state. Methemoglobin is not able to delivery oxygen because the ferric hemes of methemoglobin are unable to bind oxygen. Methemoglobin is produced physiologically as a result of deoxygenation. However, endogenous enzymatic hemoglobin reduction mechanism reduces the methemoglobin to maintain a very low steady-state blood methemoglobin level (nearly 1% of total hemoglobin). Reduction of methemoglobin back to hemoglobin is catalyzed by the (NADH)-cytochrome b5 reductase. Cytochrome b5 transfers electrons directly to methemoglobin to reduce it to hemoglobin [1].

Acyl Coenzyme A (CoA) Desaturases

Long-chain fatty acids can be synthesized endogenously in human body. Palmitate, a saturated fatty acid, is the main product of fatty acid synthase system and serves as a precursor for other long-chain fatty acids. Palmitate may be lengthened to form stearate. Palmitate and stearate are precursors of the monounsaturated fatty acids. The double bond is introduced into the fatty acid chain by an oxidative reaction catalyzed by fatty acyl-CoA desaturase. All fatty acyl-CoA desaturases are associated with both cytochrome b5 and NADH-cytochrome b5 reductase in the endoplasmic reticulum membrane [12]. Essential fatty acids are also converted to arachidonic acid by the same way.

Cytochrome p450 Family

Cytochrome p450 is a heme protein mainly localized in the smooth endoplasmic reticulum membrane. Cytochrome p450 actually is a family of closely similar proteins. Several hundred members are known. Each cytochrome p450 enzyme has a different substrate specifity. They can catalyse many types of oxidative transformations. Cytochrome p450 is responsible for metabolism of some hormones, fatty acids and detoxification of various drugs and environmental chemicals (xenobiotics) by the liver [13]. Substrates of Cytochrome p450 are generally hydrophobic and relatively insoluble. This reaction results in aliphatic or aromatic hydroxylation. Hydroxylation of substrates makes them more soluble but is more important for participation in the phase II reaction, in which a large polar group is attached to the hydroxyl oxygen by glucuronidation or sulfation. The substrate is now soluble in water and can be excreted in bile or urine. This biotransformation is protective against the harmful effects of various chemicals. However, unfortunately, hydroxylation of some foreign compounds converts them into carcinogenic or more toxic molecules. For example, benzo [α] pyrene found in cigarette smoke becomes more activated after the cytochrome p450-dependent hydroxylation during its detoxification [14].

On the other hand Cytochrome p450 is involved in the biosynthesis of cholesterol, bile acids, steroid hormones (androgens, estrogens, glucocorticoids, aldosteron) and leucotriene [1]. Cytochrome p450 of adrenal cortical mitochondria is responsible for steroid hydroxylase reactions involved in biosynthesis of 1,25 dihydroxycholecalciferol (vitamin D), and this system also contains iron-sulfur proteins.

Glutathione Peroxidase and Catalase

Reactive oxygen species, such as superoxide and hydrogen peroxide, are generated in all cells by mitochondrial and enzymatic sources as well external factors such as ionized radiation, various chemicals and drugs. These reactive species can cause oxidative damage to DNA, proteins, and membrane lipids. All cells have a defensive antioxidant system against the harmfull effects of reactive oxygen species. Glutathione peroxidase is an intracellular antioxidant enzyme. It enzymatically reduces hydrogen peroxide and organic peroxides to water to limit their harmful effects. Glutathione peroxidase is a hemoprotein containing selenium as a prosthetic group. Certain reactive oxygen species, such as hydrogen peroxide, are also essential for growth factor-mediated signal transduction, mitochondrial function, and maintenance of normal thiol redox-balance. Thus, by limiting hydrogen peroxide accumulation, glutathione peroxidase also modulates these processes [15].

Catalase is a hemoprotein containing four heme groups. It catalyzes the degredation of hydrogen peroxide. Glutathione peroxidase and catalase are present in red blood cells and other tissues and they provide an important defense against reactive oxygen and nitrogen species.

Thyroperoxidase (Iodide Peroxidase)

Thyroperoxidase, a membrane-bound heme enzyme on the luminal surface of the follicular cells in the thyroid gland. Thyroperoxidase catalyses the oxidation of iodide (I^-) that is an obligatory step in the biosynthesis of thyroid hormones. Thyroid hormones are responsible for regulation of metabolic rate. They are major regulators of production and expenditure of ATP in the body [1].

NADPH Oxidase and Myeloperoxidase

These enzymes take part in respiratory burst during the phagocytosis. Cytocidal activity of phagocytes is due to production of reactive oxygen radicals from molecular oxygen by the catalysis of NADPH oxidase. NADPH oxidase is an enzyme complex that includes a flavoprotein and cytochrome b_{558}. Majority of the oxygen consumed during the respiratory burst is converted to superoxide anion. Formation of phagolysosome is accompanied by a decrease in the pH of intracellular medium,which in turn leads spontaneous conversion of superoxide anion to hydrogen peroxide. Hydrogen peroxide is substrate for myeloperoxidase which is a heme protein present in neutrophilic granules. Myeloperoxidase catalyzes oxidation of chloride ions to hypochlorite ion. Hypochlorite ions have a powerful killing effect on bacteria [16].

Guanylyl Cyclase

The guanylyl cyclase family includes both membrane-bound and soluble isoforms expressed in nearly all cell types. Soluble isoform of guanylyl cyclase is a cytosolic protein. It is tightly associated with heme group and acts as a receptor for nitric oxide (NO), a biological messenger. NO is produced from arginine by NO synthase that is a hem containing enzyme.

NO is able to cross plasma membranes without a carrier so that diffuses into surrounding cells. In the nearby cell, it binds to the heme group of cytosolic guanylyl cyclase and leads to production of cyclic guanosine mono phosphate (cGMP). cGMP is an intracellular signal which causes to relaxation in the heart by reducing the forcefulness of contractions [17].

Tyrptophan Pyrrolase (Tryptophan 2,3-Dioxygenase)

Tyrptophan pyrrolase is an inducible iron-porphyrin enzyme of liver that catalyses oxidation of L-tryptophan to N-formyl-kynurenine. This is the first step in endogenous synthesis of nicotinic acide (vitamin B_3). Nicotinic acide is precursor in biosynthesis of NAD^+ and $NADPH^+$ [1]. NAD^+ and $NADPH^+$ are cofactors of various oxido-reductases. NAD^+ takes play in catabolic pathways, whereas $NADPH^+$ is involved in anabolic reactions.

Inorganic Iron

Other than heme form, some proteins include iron in the ionized form. Iron is present in association with inorganic sulfur atoms or with sulfur atoms of cysteine residues in the protein, or both. These proteins are named as iron-sulfur proteins. All iron-sulfur proteins participate in one-electron transfers. They are involved in fundamental biological reactions including regulation of enzyme activity, mitochondrial energy production, DNA synthesis, ribosome biogenesis, cofactor biogenesis, purine nucleotides catabolism and regulation of gene expression. At least eight iron-sulfur proteins are involved in mitochondrial electron transfer chain and take part for energy production in the body [1,18].

Approximately 65–75% of the total body iron is found in the hemoglobin of red blood cells. The liver stores 10–20% in the form of ferritin, which can be mobilized easily when needed. About 3–4% of the body's iron is present in striated muscle as an integral part of myoglobin. The rest is distributed in other tissues and used in other metabolic reactions.

IRON DEFICIENCY

As reviwed above, iron plays a pivotal role in oxygenation of tissues, production of energy, regulation of energy production and expenditure, growth, biosynthesis of vitamin B_3, immune defence, antioxidant defence and detoxification. In the case of iron deficiency, all of these functions may impair depending on severity of deficiency. Iron deficiency may a result of many overlapping factors: dietary iron deficiency; absence of compounds required for iron absorbtion (gastric acid, ascorbate); presence of compounds limiting the iron absorbtion (phytataes, tannates); lack of iron absorbtion due to disorders of gastrointestinal system; increased loss of iron due to chronic bleeding from the gastrointestinal tract or genitourinary tract, menstruation; increased demand in pregnancy and growth period or enhanced new blood production. In the initial phase of depletion of the total iron content of the body, the iron stores provide iron required for synthesis of hemoglobin and other iron-containing compounds. With exhaustion of iron stores, iron-deficiency anemia which is characterized by hypochromic and microcytic red blood cells becomes manifest, and various pathologies appear depending and not depending on anemia. Negative effect of iron deficiency on the enzymes throughout the body even without actual anemia being present had been determined many years ago [19]. As time goes, negative effects of iron deficiency in crucial organs have been clearly described.

Hormonal System and Iron Deficiency

Hormones are of four types as respect with their chemical structure: hormonal amine; peptide, protein, glycoprotein and steroid. Especially biosynthesis of peptide, protein and glycoprotein hormones is required ATP. Since cytochromes and Fe-S proteins are involved in the mitochondrial ATP production, synthesis of these hormones such as insulin, glucagon, parathyroid and pitutary hormones are indirectly effected by iron status. However, thyroid hormones are directly in relation with iron. Normal thyroid hormone status is dependent on the presence of iron. Thyroperoxidase involved in thyroid hormone synthesis is a membrane-bound heme enzyme catalyzing the two initial steps in the synthesis [20]. Sharply reduced thyroperoxidase activity in rat fed with an irone-deficient diet has been shown previously, and adverse effects of iron deficiency anemia on thyroid metabolism is attributed to decreased thyroperoxidase activity [21]. Thyroid hormones, T_3 and T_4, exert thermogenic effect. They stimulate oxygen consumption and energy expenditure by increasing ATP formation and breakdown. Thus, by increasing the ATP turnover, thyroid hormones stimulate cellular metabolic rate. Thyroid hormones exert anabolic effects in most tissues and are essential for physical growth and maturation as well mental development. They are required for nerve myelination and growth during the late fetal and early neonatal periods. In the neonatal thyroid hormone deficiency, termed as crenitism, mental retardation and growth failure occur. Thyroid hormones are also required for linear bone growth, skeletal maturation, and general somatic development during the prepubertal period. In adult, thyroid hormones increase protein synthesis in most tissues with the exception of pituitary thyrotrop. Thyroid hormones lead to tissue responsiveness to β-adrenergic stimulation by increasing the number of β-adrenergic receptors. Hypoglycemia, cold intolerance, loss of mental clearness and memory impairment observed in hypothyroidism (and also seen in iron deficiency anemia) are results of this action [1].

People in many developing countries are at high risk of both goiter and iron deficiency anemia. Especially, iron deficiency is prevalent in goitrous women and children in those countries [22,23]. Iron supplementation will be required to improve the efficacy of thyroid metabolism in areas of overlapping deficiency. Recent studies have demonstrated that a high prevalence of iron deficiency among children in areas of endemic goiter may reduce the effectiveness of iodized salt programs [22]. Therefore, iron supplementation in this areas not only to overcome anemia but also to increase the efficacy of iodine prophylaxis.

Cardiac Function and Iron Deficiency

The decreased blood hemoglobin content with increasing severity of disease in patients with chronic heart failure (CHF) was firstly documented in 2000 by Silverberg et al. [24]. Since than, various groups reported the high prevalence of anemia in patients with advanced

CHF [25-27]. Nowadays, it has been admitted that anemia confers an independent worse prognosis in patients with CHF and is relatively frequent co-morbidity in these patients. The etiology of anemia in CHF is multifactorial. Hematinic deficiencies, reduced iron uptake due to poor nutrition and malabsorption, cardiac cachexia, iron entrapment in the reticuloendothelial system, prevention of iron release from body stores, chronic renal function impairment, water retention, ACE inhibitors, angiotensine receptor blockers, acetylsalicylic acid and oral anticoagulations contribute to the development of anemia in CHF patients [28-34]. Iron deficiency plays a critical role in the anemia of CHF. In general, serum iron and ferritin levels are considered reliable markers for iron deficiency. However, it has been reported that despite seemingly adequate iron stores reflected by serum iron and ferritin levels, up to 73% of patients with advanced CHF had iron deficiency as assessed by bone marrow aspiration [35]. This data gives rise to thought that neither serum iron nor ferritin levels always reflect to iron deficiency in patients with CHF. Since ferritin is an acute phase reactant, high serum ferritin may have been derived from inflammation that accompanies the CHF.

In fact, when nutritional deficieny, malabsorption and bleedings are excluded the main cause of iron deficiency in CHF is inflammation. CHF is associated with intensified oxidative stress and activated inflammation. Inflammation can lead to inefficient iron handling and entrapment in the reticuloendothelial system resulting to inadequat serum iron level for hematopoiesis and other iron-required metabolic reactions, even in the presence of adequate total iron stores. Inflammatory cytokines produced by activated macrophages, vascular wall cells, and cardiac myocytes are elevated in CHF [36]. Certain cytokines (i.e., TNF-α, IL-6) induce hepcidin releasing from liver. Hepcidin inhibits the iron absorption from gut and blocks iron recycling from iron stores in macrophages and hepatocytes. Consequently, serum iron is decreased resulting in decreased delivery of iron to the bone marrow. Furthermore, a neverending cycle is present in inflammation; cytokines lead low iron level and low iron level leads increased cytokine production.

Iron deficiency causes severe complications in cardiac function. Anemia reduces the oxygen carrying capacity of blood so that exacerbates ischemia, impairs energy production in mitochondria in the heart and activates neurohormonal system regulating water-electrolyte balance of the body. As respect with the data obtained from animal studies, severe iron deficiency can cause both systolic and diastolic dysfunction and heart failure with pulmonary congestion, left-ventricular hypertrophy and dilation, cardiac fibrosis, proteinuria, an increase in the inflammatory cytokines and a reduction in erythropoietin levels [37]. It has been shown that rats fed with an iron-deficient diet exhibited cardiac hypertrophy characterized by aberrant mitochondrial and irregular sarcomere organization, which was accompanied by increased reactive nitrogen species [38]. Another experimental study examining the effects of anemia in a rat model of acute myocardial infarction demonstrated that anemia increases infarct size and decreases cardiac function and survival rate in acute myocardial infarction; transfusion of anemic animals up to 100 g/L Hb with fresh blood reduces infarct size and improves cardiac function [39]. In severe anemia, low Hb level leads the decreased systemic vascular resistance. Reduced systemic vascular resistance leads to low blood pressure, which in turn causes baroreceptor-mediated neurohormonal activation. Activation of sympathetic system, renin-angiotensin-aldosterone activity and vasopressin result in decreased renal blood flow and glomerular filtration rate. This situation leads to salt and water retention by the kidneys and expansion of the extracellular fluid and plasma volumes. The combined effect of volume expansion of body fluids and vasodilation increases the cardiac output that helps to increase oxygen transport [24,40]. All this can lead to left-ventricular dilation and hypertrophy, and the production and/or worsening of CHF.

Does correction of iron deficiency improve cardiac function in CHF patients? Yes, treatment with iron supplements in patients with CHF is beneficial [41,42]. A number of studies on intravenous iron supplements in anemic CHF patients have shown improved Hb level, left-ventricular ejection fraction, NYHA class, quality of life, left-ventricular hypertrophy and dilation, exercise capacity, renal function in addition to reduced heart rate decreased serum C-reactive protein and shortened hospitalization [43-45]. The improvements in cardiac function seen with correction of the iron deficiency result from a few mechanisms: 1)The improvement in anemia will reduce sympathetic, renin-angiotensin-aldosterone, and vasopressin activity and thus improve renal function, prevent increased salt/water retention and increased fluid load to the heart 2)Tachycardia alone can have a profound negative effect on cardiac function in CHF. The reduction in heart rate with correction of the anemia will reduce myocardial oxygen consumption and finally the work load of the heart, resulting a great improvement in cardiac function. 3)Another mechanism for the improvement in cardiac function is the improvement in Hb itself, which increases the oxygen supply to the heart [46,47] .

Thrombocytosis contributes to a hypercoaguable state and increases the risk of thrombosis. Thrombocytosis may occur secondary to iron deficiency. This may be explained by a few approaches: 1)Iron is a regulator of thrombopoiesis, and normal iron levels are required to prevent thrombocytosis by inhibiting thrombopoiesis 2)Reduced red cell deformability due to microcytosis is an another factor leading hypercoaguable state in iron deficiency 3)Anaemic hypoxia secondary to iron deficiency may occur in situations of increased metabolic stress such as infections, and thus the increased metabolic demands of the brain can not be met because of low hemoglobin level [48,49]. CHF is a hypercoaguable state and incidence of venous thromboembolism is greatly increased in these patients [50]. Correction of the iron deficiency may also be benefical for prevention of thrombocytosis [51].

Mental Function and Iron Deficiency

Iron is an essential element in maintaining normal structure and functions of the central nervous system. Both iron deficiency and iron overload present significant risks to the development and function of brain. The iron homeostasis in the body is maintained by liver. Hepcidin secreted by the liver coordinates iron metabolism by regulating iron absorption and reutilization in various tissues. Cells appropriately regulate iron uptake by altering expression of transferin receptor. As an exception, iron uptake by brain is out of liver-dependent macroregulatory system. Brain is separated from the systemic circulation by the blood-brain barrier which separates the central nervous system from the systemic circulation. Iron must cross an apical and basolateral membrane before it disperses to neurons [52]. In adult, brain-iron uptake is mediated by endothelial transferin receptors in the blood-brain barrier. Expression of transferrin receptors is regulated by iron content of central nervous system. Transferrin-bound iron in the systemic circulation is endocytosed by brain endothelial cells, and elemental iron is released to brain interstitial fluid by ferroportin which has been immunohistochemically detected in the blood-brain barrier [53]. A special form of the ferroxidase, ceruloplasmin is responsible for valence switch required for iron transport between compartments [54]. Transferrin is synthesized mainly by oligodendrocytes and transports iron throughout the central nervous system. Transferrin synthesized within the central nervous system does not return to the systemic circulation. After initial uptake, iron is redistributed into various areas of the brain. Once obtained, brain efficiently conserves its iron. Brain iron content decreases minimally in the severe systemic iron deficiency in human [55].

Iron deficiency occurs commonly during three phases of early life when the brain is developing: fetal life, toddlerhood and early adolescence. Iron deficiency during each time period has different effects on the central nervous system and different consequences depending on the onset, peak activity and effected brain regions [56]. Fetal and early neonatal brain iron deficiency occurs due to insufficient maternal dietary iron intake, smoking, maternal hypertension, and maternal diabetes mellitus. Maternal anemia and maternal hypertension cause restricted amount of iron to the fetus. In the case of maternal diabetes, fetal hypoxia develops leading increased erythropoiesis and enhanced iron demand [57]. All of these conditions cause decreased hepatic iron stores as reflected by highly low serum ferritin levels. Since iron is preferentially shunted to the red blood cells for hemoglobin synthesis, brain iron levels are low as 60% of normal level [58]. The neonatal serum ferritin concentration correlates with low brain iron status. Neurodevelopmental abnormalities appear at the lower ferritin concentration than 35 μg/L [59].

Neuropathology derived from iron deficiency in fetal and early neonatal time may appear as the result of a few mechanisms. Anemic hypoxia, decreased energy production due to mitochondrial dysfunction, crenitism, impaired neurotransmitter production and function, decreased polyunsaturated fatty acid concentrations in myelin and altered gene expression are the major causes of neurological abnormalities. Neurobehavioral dysfunction occur both during and after the period of deficiency. Although clinical studies are limited, animal studies on neurological abnormalities derived from fetal iron deficiency are satisfactory. Abnormalities in hippocampal dendritic structure, monoamine transmitter metabolism, and myelination have been well documented in animal models of fetal iron deficiency [60]. Formerly, neurological abnormalities derived from fetal iron deficiency were uniquely attributed to anemia and its attendant effects on cerebral oxygenation and brain metabolism. In the second half of the 1980's this opinion was changed by the documentation of reduced cytochrome c concentrations in the iron deficient brain [61]. Mitochondria are main consumers of iron in eukaryotes. The respiratory chain relies on iron-containing redox systems including iron-sulphur clusters and cytochromes. It has been discovered that iron deficiency can lead to altered cerebral energy metabolism and decreased ATP production due to reduced cytochrome c concentrations. Hippocampus that is a structure required for learning and memory is highly susceptible to iron deficiency. Iron uptake and utilization make a peak during the late fetal-early neonatal period. Iron deficiency during this period causes distinctive, long-term changes in hippocampal cellular growth and function.This can become irreversible especially in newborns, even after long-term iron supplementation [62,63].

The effect of iron deficiency on neurotransmitter production and function in the brain has been extensively carried out by Youdim et al. [64], since 1974. They have discovered that the brain striatal dopaminergic-opiate system is defective in the iron deficiency, whic in turn causes alterations in circadian behaviours, cognitive impairment and neurochemical changes.

Another major cause of neuropathology is altered fatty acid composition of the myelin. Human organism can synthesize monounsaturated fatty acids. Denovo synthesis of polyunsaturated fatty acids is impossible. Essential fatty acids are the polyunsaturated fatty acids not synthesized in the body but required for normal metabolism. Essential fatty acids are linoleic acid, linolenic acids and arachidonic acid. Linoleic acid and linolenic acid can be converted to arachidonic acid by the microsomal desaturation and chain-elognation process when the diet contains adequate amounts of lineloic acid. Microsomal fatty acyl-CoA desaturases are heme-containing enzymes. Polyunsaturated fatty acid concentrations of myelin were found to be altered in iron deficient brain [65,66].

All of the damaging effects mentioned above are ascribed to the lack of iron incorporation into functional hemoproteins and iron-sulfur proteins. Recently, it has been discovered that iron deficiency can alter the expression of some critical genes involved in development of brain, despite iron repletion. Carlson et al. [67,68] investigated the impact of late fetal-early neonatal iron deficiency on short, and long-term hippocampal gene expression. As short term changes, they have determined altered expression of genes related to hippocampal iron homeostasis, dendrite morphogenesis, synaptogenesis, and glutamatergic signaling. Genes related to protein translation and neurodegenerative processes that contribute to etiology of Alzheimer disease were also found to be altered in late fetal-early neonatal iron deficiency. The potential relation between fetal iron deficiency and Alzheimer disease was also supported by Atamna et al. [69,70]. They have reported altered expression of genes leading to beta-amyloid production, implicated in Alzheimer disease pathogenesis, in the iron deficiency during a potentially vulnerable time in hippocampal development. Furthermore, same group have taken attandance on heme's key role in the pathogenesis of Alzheimer disease. All evidences support the role of amyloid-beta peptide in the pathophysiology of Alzheimer's disease. Accumulation and aggregation of amyloid-beta peptide triggers most of the disparate cytopathologies such as loss of iron homeostasis and mitochondrial complex IV, which may initiate synaptic dysfunction, hypometabolism, and memory loss. Atamna et al. [70] have discovered that heme binds with amyloid-beta peptide , forming a complex (Abeta-heme). In this way, heme prevents the aggregation of amyloid-beta peptide. However, excessive production of Abeta-heme decreases the bioavailability of heme, resulting heme deficiency in the brain which may be a cause of mitochondrial dysfunction .

Immune Defence and Iron deficiency

Although interaction between iron status and immune defence is well described, the results of many of studies have been conflicting and hard to interpret because of variations in baseline iron status, the severity of the deficiency and the possibility of co-existing nutritional problems. Iron deficiency has been reported to be associated with increased susceptibility to infection in both human and experimental animal studies [71,72]. However, iron supplementation in humans, particularly in the tropic regions, can increase the risk of infections such as malaria and tuberculosis [71,73]. In addition, it has been reported that iron overload is also associated with increased susceptibility to infectious diseases [74]. Abnormalities of iron-dependent biochemical reactions absolutely contribute to the adverse effects of iron on the immune system. Iron requirement of the body increases during the immune response. Because; 1)The continuous generation of immune cells in bone marrow and the clonal expansion of lymphocytes in response to antigenic stimulation require the bioavailability of iron for the synthesis of deoxyribonucleotide precursors by ribonucleotide reductase which is an iron containing enzyme 2)Iron is required to maintain the activity of a number of enzymes directly involved in the immune defence processes such as respiratory burst 3) Iron contributes to activation of NF-jB which is a transcription factor required for the expression of a number of genes involved in innate immunity and inflammation [75]. Therefore deficits in iron has suppressive effects on the immune system. In the case of iron deficiency, most altered immunologic function is notably cell-mediated immunity. Majority of the human studies report decreased numbers of T lymphocytes in peripheral circulation and their decreased blastogenic response to mitogens in iron deficiency [76]. These alterations are attributed to thymic atrophy. In general, thymic atrophy is a result of increased apoptosis induced by high levels of cortisol and perhaps decreased levels of leptin. However in experimental animal studies, thymic atrophy was not found to be associated with an increase in thymocyte apoptosis in iron deficiency. Kuvibidila et al. [77] have reported that iron deficiency leads to depletion of total thymocytes without any significant differences in thymocyte subsets.

Polymorphonuclear leukocytes play essential role in host defence by the phagocytosis. Phagocytosis is the process whereby phagocytes move toward, engulf and digest foreign invaders by activation of the respiratory burst. Oxygen consumption increases 20 to 200 fold during this process. Most of the cytocidal activity of phagocytes is due to the generation of reactive oxygen species from NADPH and molecular oxygen by the reaction catalyzed by NADPH oxidase. Most of the oxygen is converted to superoxide anion, which in turn formed hydrogen peroxide by superoxide dismutase. Hydrogen peroxide is a substrate for myeloperoxidase which catalysis production of hypochlorous acid, a microbiocidal factor. Since both NADPH oxidase and myeloperoxidase are heme-containing enzymes, iron deficiency leads an impairement in phagocytosis. Decreased phagocytosis by polymorphonuclear cells in iron deficient patients has been reported [78]. Another possible cause of decreased phagocytosis may be decreased ATP production. In the case of decreased ATP production in phagocyting cells, ATPase activity decreases, which in turn leads to altered membrane fluidity and less capability to engulf foreign particles.

Iron deficiency alters the balance between pro- and anti-inflammatory cytokines, an alteration that may affect innate and cell-mediated immunity [79]. Dietary iron restriction causes a decrease in serum levels of interferon-γ, IL-12 and IL-10, which return to normal level after iron repletion. Human studies have shown decreased levels of serum IL-2 and IL-6 in iron-deficient children [80]. Pro-inflammatory cytokines such as IL-6, TNF-α and IL-1 have been shown to increase expression of hepcidin, which in turn leads to down-regulation of ferroportin on enterocytes and macrophages, and consequent inhibition of absorbtion and recycling of iron. The resultant hypoferremia is an adaptive condition due to restricting iron. Iron has a direct effect on the growth and virulence of microbial pathogens. Therefore, this important mechanism of innate anti-microbial defense is based on deprivation of an essential nutrient for pathogens. Increased risk of infections in the iron supplementation reported by Oppenheimer et al [72] may be explained by this adaptive mechanism. Chronic immune activation can lead to hypoferremia that may impair erythropoiesis. Chronic inflammatory conditions result in the development of low serum iron levels and a mild to moderate, normocytic, normochromic anemia known as the anemia of chronic disease. Hepcidin levels have been found to be elevated in inflammatory bowel disease and rheumatoid arthritis [81,82].

Conclusion

Iron deficiency is one of the most important health problem through the worldwide. Especially, it is prevalent in developing and industrialized countries. Maternal iron deficiency affects 30–50% of pregnancies and is the most common cause of newborn iron deficiency. Iron is essential for the function of all mammalian cells and contributes to various important biological processes either in the form of heme, or as inorganic iron. However iron can be cytotoxic when present at high concentrations. Intestinal absorbtion of iron is tightly regulated depending on iron status of the body. It is clear from the foregoing discussion that iron deficiency leads growth retardation, cognitive deterioration and alteration of neurological functions, decreased immune response, impaired cardiac and thyroid function. Especially, fetal- early neonatal deficiency has long-term advers effects that is implicated in the pathogenesis of Alzheimer Disease, despite the iron repletion. In this chapther, main biochemical reactions and metabolic pathways that are affected by decreased cellular iron level were reviewed. It has been aimed to give new insights into the multidirectional interaction between iron and dysfunctions in various organs.

References

[1] Bhagavan, NV. Medical Biochemistry. First edition. USA: Jones and Bartlett Publishers; 1992.

[2] Andrews, NC. Disorders of iron metabolism. *N Engl J Med*, 1999 341(26), 1986-1995.

[3] Muñoz, M; Villar, I; García-Erce, JA. An update on iron phsiology. *World J Gastroenterol*, 2009 15(37), 4617-4626.

[4] Hastka, J;Lehman, P; Weiss, G; Zawta, B. Anemia: Quesitions and Answers. First edition. Germany: Roche *Diagnostics*; 2003.

[5] Anderson, GJ; Frazer, DM. Recent advances in intestinal iron transport. *Curr Gastroenterol Rep*, 2005 7(5), 365-372.

[6] Koulaouzidis, A; Said, E; Cottier, R; Saeed, AA. Soluble transferrin receptors and iron deficiency, a step beyond ferritin. A systematic review. J Gastrointestin liver Dis, 2009 18(3), 345-352.

[7] De Domenico, I; McVey Ward, D; Kaplan, J. Regulation of iron acquisition and storage: consequences for iron-linked disorders. *Nat Rev Mol Cell Biol*, 2008 9, 72–81.

[8] Nemeth, E; Tuttle, MS; Powelson, J; Vaughn, MB; Donovan, A; Ward, DM; Ganz, T; Kaplan, J. Hepcidin regulates cellular iron efflux by binding to ferroportin and inducing its internalization. *Science*, 2004 306, 2090–2093.

[9] Knutson, MD. Iron-Sensing Proteins that Regulate Hepcidin and Enteric Iron Absorption. *Annu Rev Nutr*, 2010 30, 149-171.

[10] Nelson, D.L., and Cox, M.M.(2005). Lehninger Principles of Biochemistry: Oxidative Phosphorylation and Photophosphorylation (4. edition). New York, NY: W.H. Freeman and Company.

[11] Murray, R.K., Granner, D.K., Mayes, P.A., and Rodwell, V.W. (2000). Harper's Biochemistry: Biologic Oxidation (25. edition). Unites Stataes of America: McGraw-Hill.

[12] Enomoto, A; Omae, FM; Miyazaki, Y; Kozutsumi, T; Yubisui and A. Suzuki, Dihydroceramide:sphinganine C-4-hydroxylation requires Des2 hydroxylase and the membrane form of cytochrome b5. *Biochem J*, 2006 397, 289–295.

[13] Tompkins, LM; Wallace, AD. Mechanisms of cytochrome P450 induction. J Biochem Mol Toxicol, 2007 21(4), 176-181.

[14] Burtis, C.A., Ashwood, E.R.(Eds). (1999). Tietz Textbook of Clinical Chemistry: Liver Function (3. edition). Philadelphia, Pennsylvania: W.B. Saunders Company.

[15] Lubos, E; Loscalzo, J; Handy, DE. Glutathione peroxidase-1 in health and disease: from molecular mechanisms to therapeutic opportunities. Antioxid Redox Signal, 2010 Nov 18. [Epub ahead of print].

[16] Vlasits, J; Jakopitsch, C; Bernroitner, M; Zamocky, M; Furtmüller, PG; Obinger, C. Mechanisms of catalase activity of heme peroxidases. *Arch Biochem Biophys*, 2010 500(1), 74-81.

[17] Rudolph, V; Freeman, BA. Cardiovascular consequences when nitric oxide and lipid signaling converge. *Circ Res*, 2009 105(6), 511-522.

[18] Xu, XM; Moller, SG. Iron-sulfur clusters: Biogenesis, molecular mechanisms and their functional significance. Antioxid redox Signal, 2011 Feb 3 [Epub ahead of print].

[19] Beutler, E; Larsh, SE; Gurney, CW. Iron therapy in chronically fatigued, nonanemic women: a double-blind study. Ann Intern Med, 1960 52, 378–394.

[20] Arthur, JR; Beckett, GJ. Thyroid function. *Br Med Bull*, 1999 55(3), 658-668.

[21] Hess, SY; Zimmermann, MB; Arnold, M; Langhans, W; Hurrell, RF. Iron deficiency anemia reduces thyroid peroxidase. *J Nutr*, 2002 132(7), 1951-1955.

[22] Zimmermann, MB. The influnce of iron status on iodine utilization and thyroid function. *Annu Rev Nutr*, 2006 26, 367-389.

[23] Kandhro, GA; Kazi, TG; Afridi, HI; Kazi, N; Arain, MB; Sarfraz, RA; Sirajuddin, SN; Baig, JA; Shah, AQ. Evaluation iron in serum and urine and their relation with thyroid function in female goitrous patients. *Biol Trace Element Res*, 2008 125(3), 203-212.

[24] Silverberg, DS; Wexler, D; Blum, M; Keren, G; Sheps, D; Leibovitch, E; Brosh, D; Laniado, S; Schwartz, D; Yachnin, T; Shapira, I; Gavish, D; Baruch, R; Koifman, B; Kaplan, C; Steinbruch, S; Iaina, A. The use of subcutaneous erythropoietin and intravenous iron for the treatment of the anemia of severe, resistant congestive heart failure improves cardiac and renal function and functional cardiac class, and markedly reduces hospitalizations. *J Am Coll Cardiol*, 2000 35, 1737–1744.

[25] McClellan, WM; Flanders, WD; Langston, RD; Jurkovitz, C; Presley, R. Anemia and renal insufficiency are independent risk factors for death among patients with congestive heart failure admitted to community hospitals: a population-based study. *J Am Soc Nephrol*, 2002 13, 1928–1936.

[26] Herzog, CA; Muster, HA; Li, S; Collins, AJ. Impact of congestive heart failure, chronic kidney disease, and anemia on survival in the Medicare population. *J Card Fail*. 2004 10, 467–472.

[27] Kalra, PR; Bolger, AP; Francis, DP; Genth-Zotz, S; Sharma, R; Ponikowski, PP; Poole-Wilson, PA; Coats, AJ; Anker, SD. Effect of anemia on exercise tolerance in chronic heart failure in men. *Am J Cardiol.* 2003 91, 888–891.

[28] Witte, KK; Desilva, R; Chattopadhyay, S; Witte, KK; Desilva, R; Chattopadhyay, S; Ghosh, J; Cleland, JG; Clark, AL. Are hematinic deficiencies the cause of anemia in chronic heart failure? *Am Heart J.* 2004 147, 924-930.

[29] Anker SD, Sharma R. The syndrome of cardiac cachexia. *Int J Cardiol*, 2002 85, 51-66.

[30] Dries, DL; Exner, DV; Domanski, MJ; Greenberg B, Stevenson LW. The prognostic implications of renal insufficiency in asymptomatic and symptomatic patients with left ventricular systolic dysfunction. *J Am Coll Cardiol.* 2000 35, 681-689.

[31] Westenbrink, BD; Visser, FW; Voors, AA; Smilde, TD; Lipsic, E; Navis, G; Hillege, HL; van Gilst, WH; van Veldhuisen DJ. Anaemia in chronic heart failure is not only related to impaired renal perfusion and blunted erythropoietin production, but to fluid retention as well. Eur Heart J, 2007 28, 166-171.

[32] Weiss, G; Goodnough, LT. Anemia of chronic disease. N Engl J Med, 2005 352, 1011-1023.

[33] Ishani, A; Weinhandl, E; Zhao, Z; Gilbertson, DT; Collins, AJ; Yusuf, S; Herzog, CA. Angiotensin converting enzyme inhibitor as a risk factor for the development of anemia, and the impact of incident anemia on mortality in patients with left ventricular dysfunction. *J Am Coll Cardiol.* 2005 45, 391-399.

[34] Kaldara-Papatheodorou, EE; Terrovitis, JV; Nanas, JN. Anemia in heart failure: Should we supplement iron in patients with chronic heart failure? *Pol Arch Med Wewn*, 2010 120 (9), 354-360.

[35] Nanas, JN; Matsouka, C; Karageorgopoulos, D; Leonti, A; Tsolakis, E; Drakos, SG; Tsagalou, EP; Maroulidis, GD; Alexopoulos, GP; Kanakakis, JE; Anastasiou-Nana, MI. Etiology of anemia in patients with advanced heart failure. *J Am Coll Cardiol*, 2006 48, 2485–2489.

[36] Zhang, AS; Enns, CA. Iron homeostasis: Recently identified proteins provide insight into novel control mechanisms. J Biol Chem, 2009 284(2), 711–715.

[37] Naito, Y; Tsujino, T; Matsumoto, M; Sakoda, T; Ohyanagi, M; Masuyama, T. Adaptive response of the heart to long-term anemia induced by iron deficiency. *Am J Physiol Heart Circ Physiol*, 2009 296, H585–H593.

[38] Dong, F; Zhang, X; Culver, B; Chew, HG Jr; Kelley, RO; Ren, J. Dietary iron deficiency induces ventricular dilation, mitochondrial ultrastructural aberrations and cytochrome c release: involvement of nitric oxide synthase and protein tyrosine nitration. *Clin Sci.* 2005, 109(3), 277-286.

[39] Hu, H; Xenocostas, A; Chin-Yee, I; Lu, X; Feng, Q. Effects of anemia and blood transfusion in acute myocardial infarction in rats. *Transfusion*, 2010 50(1), 243-251.

[40] Anand, IS. Anemia and chronic heart failure. J Am Coll Cardiol, 2008 52, 501–511.

[41] Anand, IS; Chandrashekhar, Y; Ferrari, R; Poole-Wilson, PA; Harris, PC. Pathogenesis of oedema in chronic severe anaemia: studies of body water and sodium, renal function, haemodynamic variables, and plasma hormones. *Br Heart J*, 1993 70, 357– 362.

[42] Anand, IS; Chandrshekhar, Y; Wander, GS; Chawla, LS. Endothelium-derived relaxing factor is important in mediating the high output state in chronic severe anemia. *J Am Coll Cardiol*, 1995 25, 1402–1407.

[43] Bolger, AP; Bartlett, FR; Penston, HS; O'Leary, J; Pollock, N; Kaprielian, R; Chapman CM. Intravenous iron alone for the treatment of anemia in patients with chronic heart failure. *J Am Coll Cardiol*, 2006 48, 1225–1227.

[44] Usmanov, RI; Zueva, EB; Silverberg, DS; Shaked, M. Intravenous iron without erythropoietin for the treatment of iron deficiency anemia in patients with moderate to severe congestive heart failure and chronic renal insufficiency. J Nephrol, 2008 21, 236–242.

[45] Toblli, J; Lombrana, A; Duarte, P; Di Gennaro, F. Intravenous iron reduces NT-pro-brain natriuretic peptide in anemic patients with chronic heart failure and renal insufficiency. *J Am Coll Cardiol*, 2007 50, 1657–1665.

[46] Logeart, D; Gueffet, JP; Rouzet, F; Pousset, F; Chavelas, C; Solal, AC; Jondeau, G. Heart rate per se impacts cardiac function in patients with systolic heart failure and pacing: a pilot study. *Eur J Heart Fail*, 2009 11, 53–57.

[47] Fox, K; Borer, JS; Camm, AJ; Danchin, N; Ferrari, R; Lopez Sendon, JL; Steg, PG; Tardif, JC; Tavazzi, L; Tendera, M; Heart Rate Working Group. Resting heart rate in cardiovascular disease. *J Am Coll Cardiol*, 2007 50, 823–830.

[48] Balci, K; Utku, U; Asil, T; Büyükkoyuncu, N. Deep cerebral vein thrombosis associated with iron deficiency anaemia in adults. *J Clin Neurosci*, 2007 14(2), 181-184.

[49] Munot, P; De Vile, C; Hemingway, C; Gunny, R; Ganesan, V. Severe iron defi ciency anaemia and ischaemic stroke in children. *Arch Dis Child*, 2011 96, 276-279.

[50] Darze, ES; Latado, AS; Guimarães, AG; Guedes, RA; Santos, AB; de Moura, SS; Passos, LC. Incidence and clinical predictors of pulmonary embolism in severe heart failure patients admitted to a coronary care unit. *Chest*, 2005 128, 2576–2580.

[51] Dahl, NV; Henry, DH; Coyne, DW. Thrombosis with erythropoietic stimulating agents -does iron-deficient erythropoiesis play a role? *Semin Dial*, 2008 21, 210–211.

[52] Rouault, TA; Cooperman, S. Brain iron metabolism. *Semin Pediatr Neurol*, 2006 13(3), 142-148.

[53] Wu, LJ; Leenders, AG; Cooperman, S; Meyron-Holtz, E; Smith, S; Land, W; Tsai, RY; Berger, UV; Sheng, ZH; Rouault, TA. Expression of the iron transporter ferroportin in synaptic vesicles and the blood-brain barrier. *Brain Res*, 2004 1001, 108-117.

[54] Brightman, MW; Kaya M. Permeable endothelium and the interstitial space of brain. *Cell Mol Neurobiol*, 2000 20, 111-130.

[55] Beard, JL; Felt, B; Schallert, T; Burhans, M; Connor, JR; Georgieff, MK. Moderate iron deficiency in infancy: Biology and behavior in young rats. *Behav Brain Res*, 2006 170, 224-232.

[56] Thompson, RA; Nelson, CA. Developmental science and the media: Early brain development. *American Psychologist*, 2001 56(1), 5–15.

[57] Siddappa, AJ; Rao, R; Long, JD; Widness, JA; Georgieff, MK. The assessment of newborn iron stores at birth: A review of the literature and standards for ferritin concentrations. Neonatology, 2007 92, 73–82.

[58] Petry, CD; Eaton, MA; Wobken, JD; Mills, MM; Johnson, DE; Georgieff, MK. Iron deficiency of liver, heart, and brain in newborn infants of diabetic mothers. *J Pediatr*, 1992 121, 109–114.

[59] Siddappa, AM; Georgieff, MK; Wewerka, S; Worwa, C; Nelson, CA; deRegnier, R-A. Auditory recognition memory in iron-deficient infants of diabetic mothers. *Pediatric Research*, 2004 55, 1034–1041.

[60] Michael, K; Georgieff, MD. The Role of Iron in Neurodevelopment: Fetal Iron Deficiency and the Developing Hippocampus. *Biochem Soc Trans*, 2008 36(Pt 6), 1267–1271.

[61] Dallman, PR. Biochemical basis for the manifestations of iron deficiency. *Ann Rev Nutr*, 1986 6, 13–40.

[62] Rao, R; Tkac, I; Townsend, EL; Gruetter, R; Georgieff, MK. Perinatal iron deficiency alters the neurochemical profile of the developing rat hippocampus. *J Nutr*, 2003 133, 3215–3221.

[63] Ward, KL; Tkac, I; Jing, Y; Felt, B; Beard, J; Connor, J; Schallert, T; Georgieff, MK; Rao R. Gestational and lactational iron deficiency alters the developing striatal metabolome and associated behaviors in young rats. J Nutrition 2007 137, 1043–1049.

[64] Youdim, MB. Brain iron deficiency and excess; cognitive impairment and neurodegeneration with involvement of striatum and hippocampus. *Neurotox Res*, 2008 14(1), 45-56.

[65] Connor, JR; Menzies, SL. Relationship of iron to oligodendrocytes and myelination. *Glia*, 1996 17, 83–93.

[66] Beard, JL; Wiesinger, JA; Connor, JR. Pre- and postweaning iron deficiency alters myelination in Sprague-Dawley rats. Dev Neurosci, 2003 25, 308–315.

[67] Carlson, ES; Stead, JD; Neal, CR; Petryk, A; Georgieff, MK. Perinatal iron deficiency results in altered developmental expression of genes mediating energy metabolism and neuronal morphogenesis in hippocampus. *Hippocampus*, 2007 17(8), 679-691.

[68] Carlson, ES; Magid, R; Petryk, A; Georgieff, MK. Iron deficiency alters expression of genes implicated in Alzheimer disease pathogenesis. *Brain Res*, 2008 1237, 75-83.

[69] Atamna, H; Frey, WH 2nd. A role for heme in Alzheimer's disease: heme binds amyloid beta and has altered metabolism. *Proc Natl Acad Sci USA*, 2004 101(30), 11153-11158.

[70] Atamna, H. Heme binding to Amyloid-beta peptide: mechanistic role in Alzheimer's. *J Alzheimer Dis*, 2006 10(2-3), 255-266.

[71] Oppenheimer, SJ. Iron and its relation to immunity and infectious disease. *J Nutr*, 2001 131, 616S–635S.

[72] Cherayil, BJ. Iron and immunity: immunological consequences of iron deficiency and overload. *Arch Immunol Ther Exp* (Warsz), 2010 58(6), 407-415.

[73] Sazawal, S; Black, RE; Ramsan, M; Chwaya, HM; Stoltzfus, RJ; Dutta, A; Dhingra, U; Kabole, I; Deb, S; Othman, MK; Kabole, FM. Effects of routine prophylactic supplementation with iron and folic acid on admission to hospital and mortality in preschool children in a high malaria transmission setting: community-based, randomised, placebo-controlled trial. *Lancet*, 2006 367, 133–143.

[74] Gangaidzo, IT; Moyo, VM; Mvundura, E; Aggrey, G; Murphree, NL; Khumalo, H; Saungweme, T; Kasvosve, I; Gomo, ZA; Rouault, T; Boelaert, JR; Gordeuk, VR. Association of pulmonary tuberculosis with increased dietary iron. *J Infect Dis*, 2001 184, 936–939.

[75] Vallabhapurapu, S; Karin, M. Regulation and function of NfkappaB transcription factors in the immune system. *Annu Rev Immunol*, 2009 27, 693–733.

[76] Bowlus, CL. The role of iron in T cell development and autoimmunity. *Autoimmun Rev*, 2003 2(2), 73–78.

[77] Kuvibidila, SR; Porretta, C; Surendra Baliga, B; Leiva, LE. Reduced thymocyte proliferation but not increased apoptosis as a possible cause of thymus atrophy in iron deficient mice. *Br J Nutr*, 2001 86, 157 –162.

[78] Bergmann, M; Hertzel, S; Pinchasi, R; Straussberg, R; Djaldetti, M; Bessler, H. Phagocytic capacity and apoptosis of peripheral blood cells from patients with iron deficiency anemia. *Biomed Phamacother*, 2005 59, 307–311.

[79] Munoz, C; Rios, E; Olivos, J; Brunser, O; Olivares, M. Iron, copper and immunocompetence. *Br J Nutr*, 2007 98 Suppl 1, S24-28.

[80] Ekiz, C; Agaoglu, L; Karakas, Z; Gurel, N; Yalcin, I. The effect of iron deficiency anemia on function of the immune system. *Hematol J*, 2005 5, 579–583.

[81] Semrin, G; Fishman, DS; Bousvaros, A; Zholudev, A; Saunders, AC; Correia, CE; Nemeth, E; Grand, RJ; Weinstein, DA. Impaired intestinal iron absorption in Crohn's disease correlates with disease activity and markers of inflammation. *Inflamm Bowel Dis*, 2006 12, 1101–1106.

[82] Demirag, MD; Haznedaroglu, S; Sancak, B; Konca, C; Gulbahar, O; Ozturk, MA; Goker, B. Circulating hepcidin in the crossroads of anemia and inflammation associated with rheumatoid arthritis. *Intern Med*, 2009 48(6), 421-426.

In: Iron Deficiency and Its Complications
Editor: Yildiz Dincer

ISBN 978-1-61324-854-6

Chapter 4

Iron Deficiency Anemia in Gastric Surgery

Isaias Dichi[1], *José Wander Bregano*[2] *and Lúcia Helena Silva Miglioranza*[3]

[1] Department of Internal Medicine, University of Londrina, Paraná, Brazil
[2]Department of Pathology, Clinical Analysis, and Toxicology, University of Londrina, Paraná, Brazil
[3]Department of Food Science, University of Londrina, Paraná, Brazil

Abstract

Anemia is a common complication in gastric surgery. It can be caused by iron, vitamin B_{12} or folate deficiency, and its prevalence may reach up to 50% of patients. Iron deficiency anemia (IDA) is the most common form of anemia and its prevalence in gastrectomized patients varies from 15 to 54%. Independently if secondary to gastrectomy used in the treatment of peptic ulcer complications and gastric cancer or to bariatric surgery for the treatment of obesity, the main causes of IDA are reduced gastric acid secretion, duodenal exclusion, inadequate intake, rapid food passage to intestine, alkaline gastritis, and Helicobacter pylori infection in the gastric remnants. Both serum iron and ferritin levels are affected by obesity and it is difficult to compare IDA prevalence in the different kinds of bariatric surgery. Patients who will be submitted or have suffered bariatric surgery deserve a

[1] Corresponding author: Isaias Dichi, MD, PhD Address: Department of Internal Medicine. Rua Robert Koch n. 60 Bairro Cervejaria, University of Londrina. Londrina, Paraná, Brazil. CEP: 86038-440. Telephone: (55) 43 3371 2332. E-mail: dichi@sercomtel.com.br; FAX: (55) 43 3371 5100

[2] José Wander Breganó, PhD; Address: Department of Pathology, Clinical Analysis and Toxicology. Rua Robert Koch n° 60 Bairro Cervejaria, University of Londrina. Londrina, Paraná, Brazil. CEP: 86038-440 Telephone: (55) 43 3371 2200 E-mail: FAX: (55) 43 3371 2323.

[3] Lúcia Helena Siva Miglioranza, PhD Address: Department of Food Science. University of Londrina. Londrina, Paraná, Brazil. CEP: 86038-440. Telephone: (55) 43. E-mail: FAX: (55) 43.

careful analysis of iron status before diagnosing IDA. Although combining numerous parameters is considered the best way, serum transferrin receptor (sTfR) is very useful for the detection of IDA in the above conditions, because unlike ferritin, sTfR concentrations are not affected by the presence of inflammation. When sTfR is not available, there is some evidence that transferrin saturation rather than ferritin could be preferred to evaluate IDA in obese patients. Classically, ferrous sulfate has been used for iron deficiency anemia since the beginning of the 19th century. Since the 1980s, many studies have examined fortification of different foods with several others iron compounds, as ferrous glycynate, which is 2.5 to 3.4 fold more available than ferrous sulphate. In addition, it was hypothesized that iron amino acid chelates prevent iron from binding to inhibitors in food and, in deprived areas many developing countries, food is composed basically of rice, beans and vegetables, rich sources of phytates. Despite those hypothetical benefits, a clinical study has shown that ferrous sulphate had much more favorable results than ferrous chelate glycinate in gastrectomized patients with IDA. Parenteral iron treatment is recommended in those patients refractory to oral iron supplementation. More studies comparing different types of bariatric surgery are needed adding serum transferrin receptor or transferrin saturation as a tool to diagnose IDA prevalence.

1. INTRODUCTION

Peptic ulcer and its complications, such as bleeding, pyloric stenosis, and perforation, are scarce indications of gastric surgery nowadays. Thus, gastrectomy is mainly indicated in cases of gastric cancer [Mimura et al., 2008] On the other hand, the rise in the prevalence of severe obesity and co morbidities has increased dramatically bariatric surgery, which is considered the most effective treatment for this condition [Buchwald, 2005], both in developed [Bernet, 2007] and developing countries [Leonor Santos et al., 2010].

Gastrectomy and bariatric surgery can be performed by several different procedures, but all of them share iron deficiency anemia (IDA) as one of the most commonly reported nutritional complications [Papini-Berto et al., 2002; Davies, 2007]. We must have some caution in diagnosing IDA in patients submitted to bariatric surgery because obesity, as an inflammatory condition, can decrease iron and increase serum ferritin levels [Yannoff et al., 2007]. IDA etiology is multifactorial and decreased food intake, reduced iron absorption, and duodenal exclusion are considered the main causes. Therefore, IDA prevalence after gastrectomy or bariatric surgery depends, at least in part, on the altered anatomy due to the surgical procedure [Papini-Berto et al.; 2002; Kurshner, 2006].

There is also a growing evidence to support the necessity to verify IDA prior to surgery [Flancbaum et al., 2006] to assure actual IDA prevalence after surgery. Although underestimated in its importance, IDA prevention and treatment are essential, as it can be present in patients` life for more than 20 years [Tovey and Hobsley, 2000], decreasing substantially their quality of life.

In this review, despite gastric surgery is frequently performed in bariatric surgeries, we will use the term gastrectomy only for patients submitted to surgery because peptic ulcer complications or gastric cancer.

2. Gastrectomy and Bariatric Surgery Types

2.1. Gastrectomy

Gastrectomy comprises total or partial gastric surgery with duodenal (Billroth I) or jejunal (Billroth II) anastomosis (Figure 1). There is a decrease in cloridric acid and intrinsic factor secretion favoring the occurrence of IDA and vitamin B_{12} deficiency [Papini-Berto et al., 2002].

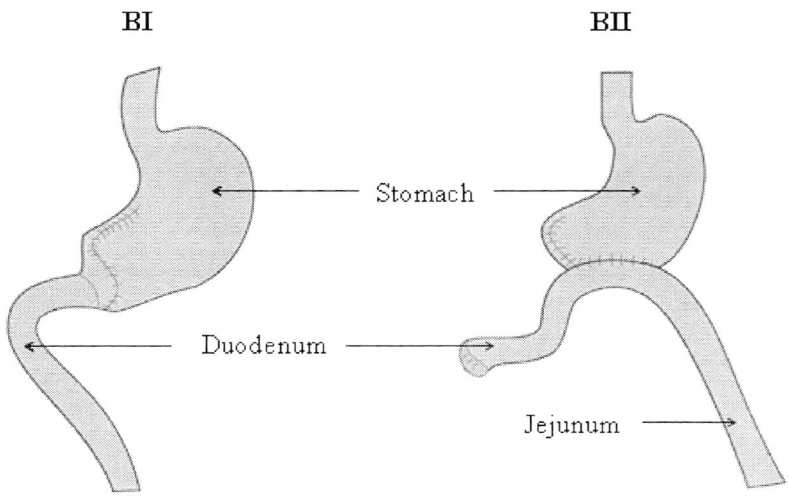

Figure 1. Gastric surgery with duodenal (Billroth I – BI) or jejunal (Billroth II - BII) anastomosis.

2.2. Bariatric Surgery

The major types of bariatric surgeries are purely restrictive procedures including vertical banded gastroplasty (VGB) and adjustable gastric banding (AGB) (Figure 2); restrictive-malabsoptive procedures (gastric bypass procedures) with predominance of restriction, such as Roux-en-Y gastric bypass (RYGB) (Figure 3), which is considered the ¨gold standard¨ procedure or with predominance of malabsorption, including biliopancreatic diversion (BPD) and BPD with duodenal switch (BPD-DS). On the other hand, purely malabsoptive procedures, which included jejunal bypass and jejunocolonic bypass, were abandoned due to the several malabsorption complications [Tucker, 2007]. Restrictive procedures basically decrease the size of the gastric reservoir, thereby decreasing the amount of food that can be consumed at one time [Shankar et al., 2010]. Thus, malabsoption of nutrients is not a concern. In contrast, restrictive-malabsorptive procedures induce weight loss through both restriction and malabsorption of food. In these bypass procedures, a portion of the small intestine, including the duodenum, is excluded from the digestive tract. A small gastric pouch is created in RYGB and is connected to a part of the jejunum (Roux limb).

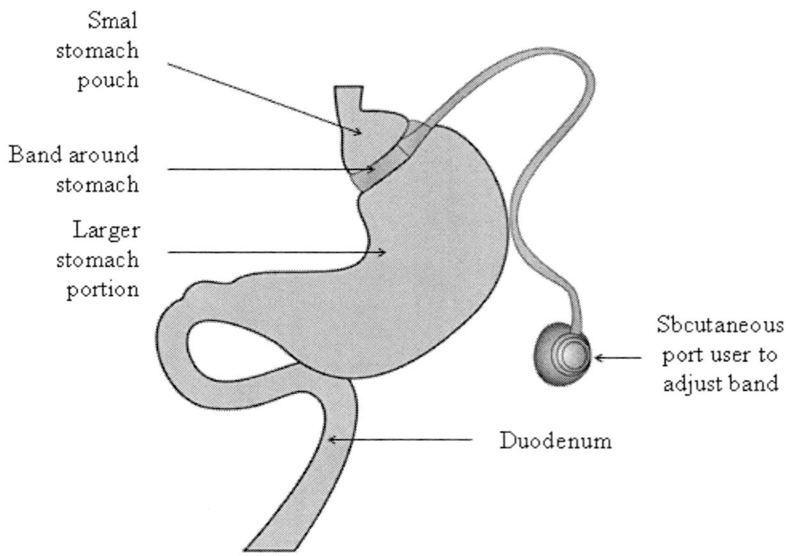

Figure 2. Adjustable gastric banding.

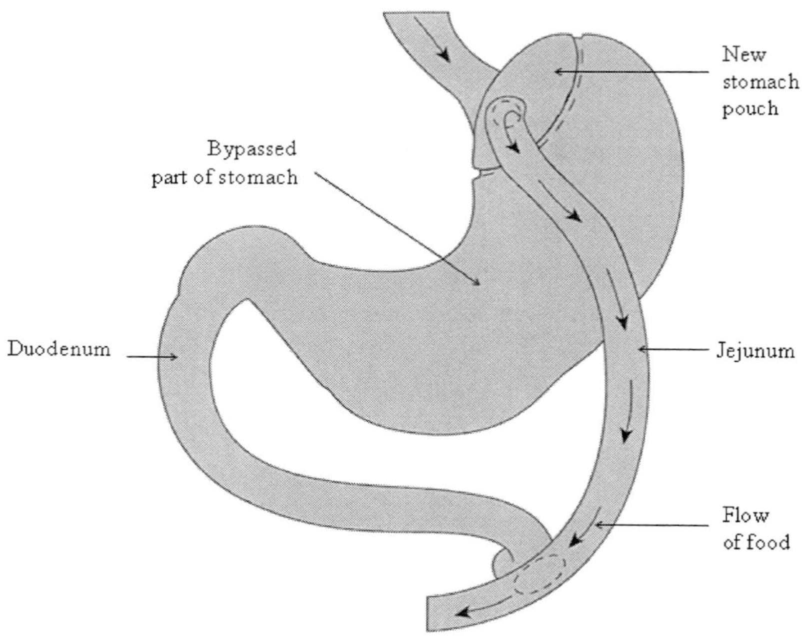

Figure 3. Roux-en-Y gastric bypass.

BPD and BPD-DS are more radical procedures, but have recently been performed more often in patients with body mass index (BMI) >50 kg/m^2 because better weight loss outcomes due to a significantly greater degree of malabsoption than RYGB, often with exclusion of the entire jejunum [Love and Billet, 2008].

Many times in super obese patients (body mass index >50 kg/m^2) a less invasive restrictive procedure can be used to achieve a degree of weight loss that will improve the general condition of the patients and permit a more effective bariatric procedure, such as RYGB, BPD or BPD-DS, to be performed later [Saber et al., 2008]. Today, every bariatric surgery procedure can be performed laparoscopically [Saber et al., 2008]. Both open and laparoscopic bariatric operations are effective therapies for morbid obesity and represent complementary procedures [Buchwald, 2005].

3. Pathophysiology Mechanisms of IDA in Gastric Surgeries

There are several reasons to explain IDA in gatrectomy and bariatric surgery, and, at least the two main pathophysiological mechanisms, decreased gastric acid secretion and duodenal exclusion, are similar in both types of surgery [Fernández-Bañares, 2009].

3.1. Reduced Food Ingestion and Avoidance of Red Meat

Reduced intake of iron-rich foods declines following gastrectomy or bypass bariatric surgeries as a result of a decrease in total caloric intake and frequent intolerance to red meat [Papini-Berto and Burini, 2001; Moize et al., 2003; Della-Costa et al. 2010]. Avinoah et al. [1992] found higher mean serum iron values in patients submitted to bypass bariatric surgery and classified as meat-eaters. They also verified chronic meat intolerance in 50% of the bypass patients. Ruz et al. [2009] performing REYGB found that meat daily consumption changed from 82.8 g meat to 55.0 g meat 18 months after 18 months.

3.2. Decreased Gastric Acid Secretion

Initial metabolism of inorganic iron (Fe^{3+}) occurs in the stomach and is facilitated by gastric acid. The solubility of inorganic iron decreases when gastric acid secretions and chloridric acid are reduced. To be absorbed, the ferric ion must be reduced to ferrous state. Consequently, ferrous iron is less absorbed in the duodenum and proximal jejunum after gastric surgery [Ukleja et al. 2004; Love et al., 2007; Mimura et al., 2008]. Both heme and non-heme iron absorption can be impaired.

Defective absorption of the heme iron contained in meat may occur, since the meat leaves the operated stomach in a poorly digested form and in quite large fragments that cannot be easily absorbed in the duodenum [Annibale et al., 2003]. Meanwhile, gastric acid secretion is considered the most important factor for the availability of non-heme iron [Annibale et al., 2003].

3.3. Duodenal Exclusion

The duodenum is excluded from digestive continuity in BII gastrectomy and any gastric bypass bariatric surgery [Papini-Berto and Burini, 2001; Love et al., 2007]. Although inorganic iron can be absorbed by the entire small intestine, most absorption of molecular iron and heme iron occurs across the apical and basolateral membranes of duodenal enterocytes. When molecular iron reaches the duodenal brush-border, it is reduced from the ferric to ferrous form by ferric reductase and transferred across the apical brush-border by the divalent metal transporter 1. Once molecular iron has been imported in the enterocyte, the body's required iron is exported into the serum through the protein ferroportin while excess iron is retained in the duodenal cell as ferritin. Therefore, exclusion of the duodenum from the digestive continuity severely impacts the body's ability to absorb [Love et al., 2007].

3.4. Rapid Food Passage to the Intestine

BII gastrectomy and any gastric bypass bariatric surgery will delay interaction of pancreatic enzymes and biliary secretions with the food bolus, and diminishes the ability to free the heme moiety from mioglobin and hemoglobin [Papini-Berto et al., 2002; Love et al., 2007].

3.5. Alkaline Gastritis and Helicobacter pylori

The increase in gastric pH due to the presence of alkaline gastritis after gastric surgery may favor the development of IDA [Mimura et al., 2008]. On the other hand, some studies have suggested a relation between *Helicobacter pylori* infection and IDA. Although multifactorial in its nature, this connection has been partially attributed to the development of alkaline gastritis due to *H. pylori* infection [Hacihanefioglu et al., 2004; Sarker et al., 2004], resulting, as a consequence, in an iron absorption disorder. The presence of *H. pylori* infection in the gastric remnants of gastrectomized patients has a high prevalence, varying from 65.1% [Onoda et al., 2001] to 80.3% [Katsube et al., 2002]. Roviello et al. [2004] found a decrease in serum levels in gastrectomized patients with *H. pylori* infection in the gastric remnant. It was also hypothesized that *H. pylori* causes IDA by competing with the host for the acquisition of alimentary iron [Annibale et al., 2003], as iron is an essential growth factor for bacteria, including *H. pylori*.

4. Diagnostic Concerns of IDA in Gastric Surgery

If combining several iron status indicators is considered the best way to assess iron status in any circumstance [Clark, 2009], it is especially true in IDA related to bariatric surgery.

Obesity may be associated with low-serum iron and high-serum ferritin concentrations, whereas metabolic syndrome (MS), a cluster of abdominal obesity, dyslipidemia, hypertension, and glucose intolerance, may be associated with high-serum ferritin concentrations. Yanoff et al. [2007]found that obese adults when compared with non-obese control subjects had lower serum iron, tranferrin saturation and mean corpuscular volume (MCV) and high significant transferrin receptor concentrations, suggesting that adiposity was associated with an increased risk for iron deficiency. By contrast, ferritin and C-reactive protein concentrations were higher in obese subjects and were positively correlated with BMI, findings consistent with the obesity status of an inflammatory condition that increases positive acute-phase reactants.

The authors concluded that the hypoferremia of obesity appeared to be explained both by true iron deficiency and by inflammatory-mediated functional iron deficiency. Della Costa et al. [2010] also verified a significant increase in the negative acute-phase reactants albumin and transferrin and a decrease in ferritin and C-reactive protein in patients submitted to bariatric surgery (RYGB) who lost 35% of their weight after one year.

On the other hand, many severely obese patients, who will be submitted to bariatric surgery, have metabolic syndrome and there is increasing evidence that this syndrome and its components are associated with serum ferritin [Zelber-Sagi et al., 2007].

In sum, patients who will be submitted or have suffered bariatric surgery deserve a careful analysis of iron status before diagnosing IDA. Although combining numerous parameters is considered the best way, serum transferrin receptor (sTfR) is very useful for the detection of IDA in the above conditions, because unlike ferritin, sTfR concentrations are not affected by the presence of inflammation [Clark, 2009]. When sTfR is not available, there is some evidence that transferrin saturation rather than ferritin could be preferred to evaluate IDA in obese patients [Coupaye et al., 2009].

5. IDA Prior to Gastric Surgery

To establish the real prevalence of IDA post gastric surgery, it is necessary, certainly, to assure that patients had not IDA prior to surgery. The etiology of patients submitted to gastrectomy (peptic ulcer complications and gastric cancer) favors the IDA high prevalence verified in these patients. However, some reports on deficiencies in parameters used to evaluate iron status prior to bariatric surgery showed an unexpected IDA high prevalence [Flancbaum et al., 2006; Schweiger et al., 2010].

Flancbaum et al. [2006] observed a prevalence of deficiency of 43.9% for iron, 22% for hemoglobin and 8.4% for ferritin, and Schweiger et al. (2010] found a prevalence of 35% for iron, 24% for ferritin, and hemoglobin and MCV low levels in 19%. Recent reports have also found an inverse relation between hemoglobin and BMI [Ernst et al., 2009; Schweiger et al., 2010], suggesting that in obese subjects micronutrient supply from consumed food could be insufficient to cover the organism`s demand [Ernest et al., 2009]. Therefore, the need to evaluate preoperative iron status is of utmost importance for the following reasons: 1st) to verify the real IDA prevalence after bariatric surgery; 2nd) to define the routine supplementation needs after bariatric surgery.

6. IDA PREVALENCE IN GASTRIC SURGERY

6.1. IDA in Total and Partial Gastrectomy and in Billroth I and Billroth II Surgeries

Although classically IDA is considered the most prevalent cause of anemia in gastrectomized patients [Meyer, 1994], some authors have mentioned that, especially with long time follow up, the more frequent type of anemia is the combination of iron and vitamin B_{12} deficiency [Tobey and Hobsley, 2000; Beyan et al., 2007; Fernadez-Bañares et al., 2009]. IDA prevalence in anemia varies from 15% to 54% in the literature [Mimura et al., 2008], however some reports have found a prevalence of IDA superior to 90% (Tobey and Hobsley, 2000; Beyan et al., 2007). The difference in the IDA prevalence between the studies could be attributed to differences in performed surgical procedures, diagnostic methods used, evaluation time and nutritional habits in the evaluated population (Beyan et al., 2007).

IDA has higher prevalence and is more precocious and severe after total gastrectomy than after partial gastrectomy (Papini-Berto et al., 2002). The influence of evaluation time can be seen in the paper by Tobey and Hobsley [2000] who followed up a gastrectomy population of 227 patients during 30 years. The authors found an IDA increase from 31.5% to 67.5% in male, and from 61.3% to 91.7% in female after 10 and 30 years, respectively.

Although theoretically due to duodenal exclusion, Billroth II could be expected to have a higher IDA prevalence than Billroth I procedure, it does not have occurred [Tobey and Hobsley, 2000; Annibale et al., 2003].

6.2. IDA in Bariatric Surgery

6.2.1. Roux-en-Y Gastric Bypass: the Gold Standard Procedure

REYGB is a primarily restrictive procedure with a mild component of malabsorption [Fujioka, 2005]. In this procedure, gastric capacity is reduced by 90-95% [Alvarez-Leite, 2004]. REYGB has shown highly satisfactory results in weight loss, improvement of medical conditions and long-term quality of life [Ruz et al., 2009]. The postoperative mortality rate associated with this technique is low [Buchwald et al., 2007]. IDA is one of the most prominent findings in REYGB, particularly in menstruating women [Xanthakos et al., 2006]. The size of gastric pouch left after gastric bypass is 15-20 mL. This has important effects on iron digestion because gastric juice allows not only for iron releases from its protein matrix but also solubilization and ionization of dietary iron. It also contributes to maintain iron on its reduced form [Ruz et al., 2009]. Besides, duodenal and proximal jejunum, the main areas of iron absoption, are bypassed [Alvarez-Leite, 2004].

Although not exclusively, IDA prevalence depends significantly on time evaluation. After one year, Toh et al. [2009] verified a significant increase in patients with low serum ferritin iron from 2% to 15% and in the overall prevalence of anemia from 6.2% to 17.2%, whereas Della Costa et al. [2010} showed a significant reduction in serum ferritin, especially in women, with a concomitant decrease in hemoglobin levels. Vargas-Ruiz et al. [2008], performing laparoscopic REYGB found that IDA prevalence varied from 20% to 36.3% after 2 and 3 years, respectively. Ruz et al. [2009] evaluated the effects of REYGB on iron status and iron absorption at different stages after surgery. They verified that the percentage of the anemic subjects changed from 1.5% at the beginning of the study to 38.8% at 18 months. The proportion of patients with low serum ferritin increased from 7.5% to 37.3%. The prevalence of IDA was 23.9% at the end of the study. Iron absorption decreased significantly after 6 months from around 40% of their initial values.

6.2.2. Restrictive Procedures

Although gastric bypass is currently considered the most popular procedure performed in the United States and worldwide [Buchwald, 2005], most European surgeons preferred a less invasive surgery, such as gastric banding until few years ago [Biertho et al., 2003]. Gastric banding is the least invasive of the purely restrictive bariatric surgery procedures. It consists of the creation of a small upper gastric pouch with restricted orifice to the rest of the stomach. This surgery limits the amount of food the stomach can hold and slow the rate of gastric emptying. It is feasible by gastroplasty or laparoscopically. Since there is no rerouting of the intestine, the risk for developing micronutrient deficiencies is entirely dependent on the patient s diet and eating habits [Buchwald, 2005; Kushner, 2006]. Although the risk of IDA is smaller compared with REYGB, the weight loss in these techniques is, in general, less than the established as the criterion of success (excess weight loss > 50% sustained for at least 5 years after surgery [Alvarez-Leite, 2004]. In contrast, Biertho et al. [2003] reported that both laparoscopic adjustable gastric banding and laparoscopic gastric bypass (LGB) provided an excess weight loss above 50%, but this criterion was met faster after LGB (6 months versus 24 to 36 months), and excess weight loss was 10% to 20% superior in the LGB group.

Giusti et al. [2004] found low iron levels in 35% of patients before surgery, but no significant change was observed during the first 12 months after laparoscopic gastric banding. After the second year of follow-up, although significant differences in mean serum iron or ferritin levels were not observed, they verified, in a multivariate analysis, that those patients who had a significant decrease in hemoglobin had also a significant decrease in serum iron levels [Gasteyger et al., 2006].

More recently, sleeve gastrectomy has reemerged as another restrictive procedure. It involves removing the fundus and greater portion of the stomach, leaving a lesser curvature tube. As ghrelin, a potent orexigenic hormone is mainly synthesized in the gastric fundus, the levels of ghrelin should be altered and this factor could increase weight loss in this procedure [Melissas et al., 2007; Melissas et al., 2008]. Studies on micronutrient deficiencies after sleeve gastrectomy are still scarce [Gherer et al., 2010).

6.2.3. Comparison between Bariatric Surgery Procedures

6.2.3.1. Roux-en-Y Gastric Bypass versus Purely Restrictive Procedures

Kalfarentzos et al. [2006] compared vertical banded gastroplasty (VBG) and REYGB in a non-superobese (BMI < 50 kg/m^2) population. They verified at 5th year follow-up, anemia prevalence in 38% and 47%, and low serum iron levels in 27% and 39% in patients submitted to REYGB and VGB, respectively. All premenopausal women in REYGB group of patients received 80 mg of iron daily, and this routine supplementation certainly explain the unexpected higher prevalence in anemia and low serum iron in patients submitted to VGB compared with REYGB. Gherer et al. [2010] also compared laparoscopic sleeve gastrectomy (LSG) and laparoscopic REYGB. They verified low serum iron levels in 18% after LSG and 28% after laparoscopic REYGB. Sleeve gastrectomy allows food passing faster through the upper gastrointestinal tract but still coming into contact with the antrum, duodenum, and proximal jejunum and this can justify the lower serum iron decrease prevalence in sleeve gastrectomy compared with gastric bypass surgeries. Ledoux et al. [2006] also verified that REYGB was more efficient than adjustable gastric banding (AGB) in correcting obesity, but that operation was associated with a higher frequency of hemoglobin decrease. The authors expanded their observation about IDA in bariatric surgery three years later [Coupaye et al., 2009] and found that hemoglobin concentrations were correlated to iron parameters, but not to vitamin B12 and folate concentrations. Moreover, hemoglobin concentrations were better correlated to serum iron and transferrin saturation than to ferritin. Serum ferritin concentrations were dependent not only of iron status but also of other parameters such as markers of inflammation, markers of insulin resistance and alanine aminotransferase, a marker of liver steatosis. Taken together, the results suggest that serum ferritin is not a good marker in this specific population.

6.2.3.2. REYGB versus Biliopancreatic Diversion Procedures

Skroubis et al. [2002] compared REYGB performed in morbidly obese patients and REYGB associated with biliopancreatic diversion (BPD) procedure in superobese patients. They found a significant increase in the percentage with low serum ferritin levels in patients submitted to REYGB (37.7%) compared with REYGB and BPD (15.2%). Of note, the incidence of hemoglobin, serum iron, and ferritin deficiency increased with time in both group of patients, around 40-50% after 4 years. Then, four years later, the same group (Skroubis et al., 2006) compared the same two procedures above in a non-superobese population (BMI between 35 and 50 kg/m^2). Weight loss after REYGB and BPD was consistently greater than after REYGB. They found that anemia was present in 33% of REYGB patients and in 40% of REYGB and BPD patients after two years. Decreased serum iron levels were seen in 20% of patients in both groups and low ferritin levels were verified in 25.9% of REYGB and BPD and in 14.6% of REYGB patients. Aasheim et al. [2009] compared laparoscopic REYGB with laparoscopic BPD with duodenal switch (BPD-DS) in superobese patients. Although after BPD-DS procedure, patients had a lower BMI than after REYGB (mean reduction 41% compared with 30%), they had more nutrient deficiencies shown by various fat-soluble (vitamins A and D) and water-soluble (thiamin) vitamins and also by a lower mean hemoglobin concentration throughout all the study (measures at 6 weeks, 6 months and one year).

6.2.3.3. Biliopancreatic Diversion with versus Biliopancreatic Diversion without Duodenal Switch

Marceau et al. [1998] compared patients receiving BPD, which excludes the duodenum, with those receiving BPD-DS, which may maintain some duodenal function. They found that those with duodenal switch had a significant higher serum ferritin levels and also a significantly lower prevalence of patients who showed decreased serum iron and ferritin levels. On the other hand, Dolan et al. [2004] found no differences in terms of weight loss or nutrient deficiencies between the procedures and an overall percentage of 32.5% anemic patients after 3 years, and concluded that there were no additional advantages in BPD with duodenal switch procedure over BPD without duodenal switch.

7. Prevention and Treatment of IDA after Gastric Surgery

Although multivitamins supplements are routinely recommended as prophylaxis against nutritional and metabolic complications in gastric surgery, they do not consistently protect patients from specific deficiencies [Brolin et al., 1998; Papini-Berto et al., 2002; Mason et al., 2005; Gasteyger et al., 2008]. Gasteyger et al. [2008] suggested the development of a ¨multi-pill¨ or injection containing appropriate doses of vitamin B12, iron, calcium and vitamin D, and folic acid or a rigorous post-operative follow-up to detect precociously the above most frequent deficiencies.

As menstruating women are more prone to IDA after gastric surgery, 320 mg of ferrous sulfate capsules twice daily, containing a total of 100 mg of elemental iron, may be prescribed for all of them [Brolin et al. 1998; Mason et al., 2005; Love et al., 2007]. It is required at least 4 months to correct iron stores in IDA (Love et al., 2007). Patients ongoing follow-up adequately, with multivitamins and additional supplementation for the corresponding deficiency, have their post operative percentage of abnormal vitamins and micronutrient levels decreased to insignificant rates [Madan et al., 2006]. An outstanding percentage of IDA occurs with time, reaching 91.7% in female, but still affecting 67.5% in male after 30 years (Tobey and Hobsley, 2000). Therefore, if men and post menopausal women are not immediately submitted to the same prevention procedures like pre menopausal women are, they must be followed-up at 6-month intervals.

Although iron is better absorbed between meals, for practical reasons to avoid their side effects, such as nausea, epigastric discomfort, abdominal cramps, and constipation, it must be given during meals. Also, vitamins C and A, enhancers of iron absorption [Rhode et al., 1998; Ahmed, 2001], must have their ingestion stimulated during meals, especially in patients with meat intolerance. Excessive amounts of iron-absoption inhibitors, such as tea, bran, cereal, and calcium-rich foods should be avoided along with ingestion of iron supplements. Although calcium may interfere with iron absorption, in long-term fortification studies this influence decreased or ceased after 3 months [Miglioranza et al., 2003], as mature cells in the presence of a continuous supply of iron are stimulated to produce high-affinity proteins, resulting in more efficient iron absorption by the enterocytes [Minihane and Fairweather-Trait, 1998]. It is unknown whether the same behavior would occur with calcium-rich foods and iron supplements instead of iron food fortification. Iron-absorption inhibitors also include drugs that reduce stomach acid level, such as antiacids, histamine H2-receptor antagonists, proton pump inhibitors, etc. [McColl, 2009].

Since the 1980s, many studies have examined fortification of different foods with several others iron compounds, as ferrous glycynate, which is 2.5 to 3.4 fold more available than ferrous sulphate. In addition, it was hypothesized that iron amino acid chelates prevent iron from binding to inhibitors in food and, in deprived areas many developing countries, food is composed basically of rice, beans and vegetables, rich sources of phytates [Miglioranza et al., 2003]. Despite those hypothetical benefits, a clinical study from Brazil [Mimura et al., 2008], where staple food is rice and beans, has shown the superiority of ferrous sulfate over ferrous chelate glycinate. They found that patients with IDA after gastrectomy treated with ferrous sulfate presented better results in all mean hematologic laboratory parameters compared to those who used ferrous chelate glycinate. After 4 months, only one patient (1/9) using ferrous sulfate had IDA in contrast to six patients (6/9) using ferrous glycinate.

Patients who remain refractory to oral supplementation or are non compliant with their oral supplementation require parenteral iron treatment, especially those with hemoglobin levels below 10 g/dL [Love et al., 2007].

Conclusion

All physicians should know the potential nutritional and metabolic problems of patients submitted to gastrectomy or bariatric surgery and help to diagnose, prevent, and treat them for the entire duration of patients` life [Mason et al., 2005; Love et al., 2007]. REYGB seems to be the preferable surgery, because it combines higher weight loss than purely restrictive patients with lower fat soluble deficiencies than BPD with or without DS. The combination of several parameters (HB, transferrin saturation, ferritin levels) is always preferable to detect IDA. Whereas IDA diagnosis before or after gastrectomy is not a difficult task, the same does not apply to IDA before or after bariatric surgery. As the majority of reports on IDA in bariatric surgery are based on serum iron and ferritin levels and both parameters are affected by obesity, it is difficult to compare IDA prevalence in the different kinds of bariatric surgery. Moreover, ferritin is associated with insulin resistance, and many of the obese patients have concomitantly metabolic syndrome. Serum transferrin receptor, when available or transferrin saturation must be added as a fundamental tool to make reliable diagnoses of IDA in bariatric surgery. Menstruating women may receive iron supplements to prevent IDA in gastric surgery. Men and post menopausal women can be followed-up at 6 months intervals. All patients must receive multivitamins after surgery, although monitoring is mandatory on account of the development of specific deficiencies (iron, vitamin B12, folic acid, calcium and vitamin D, thiamin, fat soluble vitamins), many of them depending on the surgery procedure. Ferrous sulfate continues to be the first oral choice to treat IDA. A comprehension about inhibitors and enhancers of iron absorption is helpful to avoid excessive consumption of the former (tea, coffee, chocolate, bran, cereals, milk and milk derived products, antiacids, histamine H2-receptor antagonists, proton pump inhibitors, etc) and stimulate consumption of the later (vitamin C, vitamin A). Patients who remain refractory to oral supplementation or are non compliant with their oral supplementation require parenteral iron treatment. More studies comparing different types of bariatric surgery are needed adding serum transferrin receptor or transferrin saturation as a tool to diagnose IDA prevalence.

References

AAsheim, E.T.; Björkman, S.; Sovik, T.; Engström, M.; Hanvold, S.E.; Mala, T. Olbers, T.; Bohmer, T. (2009). Vitamin status after bariatric surgery: a randomized study of gastric bypass and duodenal switch. *Am J Clin Nutr*, 90, 15-22.

Ahmed, F.; Khan, M.R.; Jackson, A. A. (2001). Concomitant supplemental vitamin A enhances the response to weekly supplemental iron and folic acid in anemic teenagers in urban Bangladesh. Am J Clin Nutr, 7, 108-115.

Alvarez-Leite, J.I. (2004). Nutrient deficiencies secondary to bariatric surgery. *Curr Opin Clin Nutr Metab Care*, 7, 569-575.

Annibale, B.; Capurso, G.; Delle Fave, G. (2003). The stomach and iron deficiency anemia: a forgotten link. *Digestive and Liver Disease*. 35, 288-295.

Avinoah, E.; Ovnat, A.; Charuzi, I. (1992) Nutritional status seven years after Roux-En-Y gastric bypass surgery. *Surgery,* 111, 137-42.

Bernett, C.P.; Ciangura, C.; Coupaye, M.; Czernichow, S.; Bouillot, J.L.; Basdevant, A. (2007). Nutritional deficiency after gastric bypass: diagnosis, prevention and treatment. *Diabetes &and Metabolism*, 33, 13-24.

Beyan, C; Beyan, E; Kaptan, K; Ifran, A; Uzar, A.I. (2007). Post-gastrectomy anemia: evaluation of 72 cases with post-gastrectomy anemia. *Hematology*, 12, 81-84.

Biertho, L.; Steffen, R.; Ricklin, T.; Horber, F.F.; Pomp, A.; Inabnet, W.B.; Herron, D.; Gagner, M. (2003). Laparoscopic gastric bypass versus laparoscopic adjustable banding: a comparative study of 1200 cases. *J Am Coll Surg*, 197, 536-547.

Brolin, R.E.; Gorman, J.H.; Gorman, R.C.; Petschenik, A.J.; Bradley, L. S.; Kenler, H.A.; Cody, R.P. (1998). Prophylactic iron supplementation after Roux-en-Y gastric bypass. *Arch Surg,* 133, 740-744.

Buchwald, H. (2005). Bariatric surgery for morbid obesity: Health implications for patients, health professionals, and third-party payers. *J Am Coll Surg*, 200, 593-604.

Buchwald, H.; Estok, R.; Fahrbach, K; Banel, D.; Sledge, I. (2007). Trend in mortality in bariatric surgery: a systematic review and meta-analysis. *Surgery*, 142, 621-635.

Clark, S.F. (2009). Iron deficiency anemia: diagnosis and management. *Curr Opin Gastroenterol*, 25, 122-128.

Coupaye, M.; Puchaux, K.; Bogard, C.; Msika, S.; Jouet, P.; Clerici, C.; Larger, E.; Ledoux, S. (2009). Nutritional consequences of adjustable gastric banding and gastric bypass: a 1-year prospective study. *Obes Surg*, 19, 56-65.

Davies, D.J.; Baxter, J.M.; Baxter, J.N.(2007). Nutritional deficiencies after bariatric surgery. *Obes Surg*, 17, 1150-1158.

Della Costa, L..; Valezi, A.C.; Matsuo, T.; Dichi, I.; Dichi, J.B. (2010). Nutritional and metabolic evaluation of patients after one year of gastric bypass surgery. *Rev Col Bras Cir*, 37, 96-101. (in Portuguese).

Dolan, K.; Hatzifotis, M.; Lowe, N.; Fielding, G. (2004). A clinical nutritional comparison of biliopancreatic diversion with and without switch. *Ann Surg*, 240, 51-56.

Ernst, B.; Thurnheer, M.; Schmid, S.M.; Schultes, B. (2009). Evidence for the necessity to systematically assess micronutrient status prior to bariatric surgery. *Obes Surg*, 19, 66-73.

Fernández-Bañares, F.; Monzón, H.; Forné, M. (2009). A short review of malabsorption and anemia. *WJG*, 15, 4644-4652.

Flancbaum, L.; Belsley, S.; Drake, V.; Colarusso, T.; Tayler, E. (2006). Preoperative nutritional status of patients undergoing Roux-en-Y gastric bypass for morbid surgery. *J Gastrointest Surg*, 10, 1033-1037.

Fujioka, K. (2005). Follow-up op nutritional and metabolic problems after bariatric surgery. *Diabetes Care*, 28, 481-484.

Gasteyger, C.; Suter, M.; Calmes, J.M.; Gaillard, R.C.; Giusti, V. (2006). Changes in body composition, metabolic profile and nutritional status 24 months after gastric banding. *Obes Surg*, 16, 243-250.

Gasteyger, C.; Suter, M.; Gaillard, R.C.; Giusti, V. (2008). Nutritional deficiencies after Roux-en-Y gastric bypass for morbid obesity often cannot be prevented by standard multivitamin supplementation. *Am J Clin Nutr*, 87, 1128-1133.

Gehrer, S.; Kern, B.; Peters, T.; Christoffel-Courtin, C.; Peterly, R. (2010) Fewer nutrient deficiencies after laparoscopic sleeve gastrectomy (LSG) than aftet Laparoscopic Roux-Y-gastric bypass (LRYGB) – a prospective study. *Obes Surg*, 20:447-453.

Giusti, V.; Suter, M.; Gaillard, R.C.; Burckhardt, P. (2004). Effects of laparoscopic gastric banding on body composition, metabolic profile and nutritionsl status of obese women: a 12-months follow-up. *Obes Surg*, 14, 239-245.

Hacihanefioglu, A.; Edebali, F.; Celebi, A.; Karakaya, T.; Senturk, O.. Hulagu, S. (2004). Improvement of Complete Blood Count in Patients with Iron Deficiency Anemia and Helicobacter pylori Infection after the eradication of Helicobacter pylori. *Hepatogastroenterology*, 51, 313-315.

Kalfarentzos, F.; Skroubis, G.; Kehagias, I.; Mead, N.; Vagenas, K. (2006). A prospective comparison of vertical banded gastroplasty and Riux-en-Y gastric bypass in a non-siperobese population. *Obes Surg*, 16, 151-158.

Katsube, T.; Ogawa, K.; Hamaguchi, K.; Murayama, M.; Konnno, S.; Shimakawa, T.; Naritaka, Y; Yagawa, H.; Kajiwara, T. (2002) Aiba M. Prevalence of Helicobacter pylori in the Residual Stomach after Gastrectomy after Gastric Cancer. *Hepatogastro-enterology*, 49, 128-132.

Kushner, R.F. (2006). Micronutrient deficiencies and bariatric surgery. *Curr Opin Endocrinol Diabetes* 13, 405-411.

Ledoux, S.; Msika, S.; Moussa, F.; Larger, E.; Boudou, P.; Salomon, L.; Roy, C.; Clerici, C. (2006). Comparison of nutritional consequences of conventional therapy of obesity, adjustable gastric bamding, and gastric bypass. *Obes Surg* 16, 1041-1049.

Love, A.L.; Billet, H.H. (2008). Obesity, bariatric surgery, and iron deficiency: True, true, true and related. *Am J Hematol*, 83, 403-409.

Madan, A.K.; Orth, W.S.; Tichansky, D.S..; Ternovits, C.A. Vitamin and trace mineral levels after laparoscopic gastric bypass. *Obes Surg*, 16, 603-606.

Marceau, P; Hould, F.S.; Simard, S.; Lebel, S.; Bourque, R.A..; Potvin, M.; Biron, S. (1998). Biliopancreatic diversion with duodenal switch. World J Surg, 22, 947-954.

Mason, E.; Jalagani, H., Vinik, A.I. (2005). Metabolic complications of bariatric surgery: diagnosis and management issues. *Gastornterol Clin North Am*, 34, 25-33.

McColl, K.E. (2009). Effect of proton pump inhibitors on vitamins and iron. *Am J Gastroenterol*, 104, suppl 2, S5-S9.

Melissas, J.; Daskalakis, M.; Koukoraki, S.; Askoxylakis, J.; Metaxari, M.; Dimitriadis, E.; Stathaki, M.; Papapdakis, J.A. (2008). Sleeve gastrectomy – a ¨Food Limiting¨ operation. *Obes Surg*, 18, 1251-1256.

Melissas, J.; Koukoraki, S.; Askoxylakis, J.; Stathaki, M.; Daskalakis, M.; Perisinakis, K.; Karkavitsas, N. (2007). Sleeve gastrectomy – a restrictive procedure? *Obes Surg*, 17:57-62.

Meyer, J.H. (1994). Nutritional outcomes of gastric surgery. *Gastroenterol Clin North Am,* 23, 227-260.

Miglioranza LHS, Matsuo T, Caballero-Córdoba GM, Dichi JB, Cyrino ES, Oliveira IBN, Martins MS, Polezer NM &and Dichi I. (2003). Effect of long-term fortification of whey drink with ferrous bysglicinate on anemia prevalence in children and adolescents from deprived areas in Londrina, Paraná, Brazil. *Nutrition*, 19, 419-421.

Mimura, E.C.M.; Breganó, J.W.; Dichi, J.B.; Gregório, E.P.; Dichi, I. (2008). Comparison of ferrous sulfate and ferrous glycinate chelate for the treatment of iron deficiency anemia in gastrectomized patients. *Nutrition*, 24, 663-668.

Minihane, A.M.; Fairweather, S.J. (1998). Effect of calcium supplementation on daily nonheme-iron absorption and long-term iron status. *Am J Clin Nutr*, 68, 96-102.

Moize, V.; Geliebter, A.; Gluck, M.E.; Yahav, E.; Lorence, M.; Coralusso, T.; Drake, V.; Flancbaum, L. (2003). Obese patients have inadequate protein intake related to protein intolerance up to 1 year following Roux-en-Y gastric bypass. *Obes Surg*, 13, 23-28.

Onoda, N.; Maeda, K.; Sawada, T.; Wakasa, K.; Arakawa, T.; Chung, K.H.Y.S. Prevalence of Helicobacter pylori infection in gastric remnant after distal gastrectomy for primary gastric cancer. *Gastric Cancer* 2001; 4: 87-92.

Papini-Berto, S.J.; Burini, RC. (2001). Causes of malnourishment in post-gastrectomized patients. *Arq Gastroenterol,* 38, 272-275. (in Portuguese).

Papini-Berto, S.J.; Maio, R.; Modolo, A.K.; dos Santos, M.D.B.; Dichi, I.; Burini, R.C. (2002). Protein-energy deficiency in gastrectomized patients. *Arq Gastroenterol*, 39, 3-9. (in Portuguese).

Rhode, B.M.; Shustik, C.; Chritou, N.V. (1999). Iron absorption and therapy after gastric btpass. *Obes Surg*, 9:17-21.

Roviello, F.; Fotia, G.; Marrelli, D.; De Stefano, A.; Macchiarelli, R.; Pinto, E. (2004). Iron deficiency anemia after subtotal gastrectomy for gastric cancer. *Hepatogastroenterology*, 51, 1510-1514.

Ruz, M.; Carrasco, F.; Rojas, P.; Codoceo, J.; Inostroza, J.; rebolledo, A.; Basfi-fer, K.; Csendes, A; Papapietro, K.; Pizarro, F.; Olivares, M.; Sian, L.; Westcott, J.L.; Hambidge, M.H.; Krebs, N.F. (2009). Iron absorption and iron status are reduced after Roux-en-Y gastric bypass. *Am J Clin Nutr*, 90, 527-532.

Saber, A.A.; Elgamal M.H.; McLeod, M.K. (2008). Bariatric surgery: the past, present, and future. *Obes Surg*, 18, 121-128.

Santos, LMP; Oliveira, IV; Peters, LR; Conde, WL. (2010). Trends in morbid obedity and in bariatric surgeries covered by the Brazilian Public Health System. *Obes Surg*, 20, 943-948.

Sarker, S.A.; Davidsson, L.; Mahmud, H.; Walczyk, T.; Hurrell, R.F.; Gyr, N.; Fuchs, G.J. (2004). Helicobacter pylori infection, iron absorption, and gastric acid secretion in Bangladeshi children. *Am J Clin Nutr*, 80, 149-153.

Schweiger, C.; Weiss, R.; Berry, E.; Keidar, A. (2010). Nutritional deficiencies in bariatric surgery candidates. *Obes Surg*, 20, 193-197.

Shankar, P.; Boylan, M.; Sriram, K. (2010). Micronutrient deficiencies after bariatric surgery. *Nutrition* 26, 1031-1037.

Skroubis, G.; Anesidis, S.; Kehagias, I.; Mead, N.; Vagenas, K.; Kalfarentzos, F. (2006). Roux-en-Y gastric bypass versus a variant of biliopancreatic diversion in a non-superobese population: a prospective comparison of the efficacy and the incidence of metabolic deficiencies. *Obes Surg*, 16, 488-495.

Skroubis, G.; Sakellaropoulos, G.; Pouggouras, K.; Mead, N.; Nikiforidis, G.; Kalfarentzos, F. (2002). Comparison of nutritional deficiencies after Roux-en-Y gastric bypass and after biliopancreatic diversion with Roux-en-Y gastric bypass. *Obes Surg*, 12, 551-558.

Toh, S.T.; Zarshenas, N.; Jorgensen, J. (2009). Prevalence of nutrient deficiencies in bariatric patients. *Nutrition*, 25, 1150-1156.

Tovey, FI; Hobsley, M. (2000). Post-gastrectomy patients need to be followed up for 20-30 years. *WJG*, 6, 45-48.

Tucker, O.N.; Szomstein, S.; Rosenthal, R.J. (2007). Nutritional consequences of weight-loss surgery. *Med Clin N Am,* 91, 499-514.

Ukleja, A.; Stone, R.L. (2004). Medical and gastroenterologic management of the post-bariatric surgery patient. *J Clin Gastroenterol*, 38, 312-321.

Vargas-Ruiz, A.G.; Hernández-Rivera, G.; Herrera, M.F. (2008) Prevalence of iron, folate, and vitamin B12 deficiency anemia after laparoscopic Roux-en-Y gastric bass. *Obes Surg*, 18, 288-293.

Xanthakos, S.A.; Inge, T.H. (2006). Nutritional consequences of bariatric surgery. *Curr Opin Clin Nutr Metab Care*, 9, 489-496.

Yanoff, L.B.; Menzie, C.M.; Denkinger, B.; Sebring, N.G.; McHugh, T.; Remaley, A.T.; Yanovski, J.A. (2007). Inflammation and iron deficiency in the hypoferremia of obesity. *International Journal of Obesity*, 31, 1412-1419.

Zelber-Sagi, S; Nitzan-Kaluski, D.; Halpern, Z; Oren, R. (2007). NAFLD and hyperinsulinemia are major determinants of serum ferritin levels. *J Hepatol*, 46, 700-707.

In: Iron Deficiency and Its Complications
Editor: Yildiz Dincer
ISBN 978-1-61324-854-6

Chapter 5

Fortification of Food with Iron: Old and New Strategies

Lúcia Helena Silva Miglioranza[4], *José Wander Bregano*[5] *and Isaias Dichi*[6]

[1]Department of Food Science and Technology, University of Londrina, Paraná, Brazil
[2]Department of Pathology, Clinical Analysis, and Toxicology, University of Londrina, Paraná, Brazil
[3]Department of Internal Medicine, University of Londrina, Paraná, Brazil

Abstract

Iron deficiency (ID) is the most common nutritional deficiency disorder in the world, affecting more than two billion people, mostly infants, children and women of childbearing age. In general, iron deficiency symptoms are attributed due to an insufficient supply of iron to the tissues, and probably not to lowered hemoglobin level. The human brain develops up until to about 20 years of age, and brain iron content also increases concomitantly up to this age. It may be difficult to repair negative effects of ID developed during this period. Several reviews and recent reports show negative effects of ID related to mental symptoms in infants and children, but unrelated to anemia; even in adolescents there exist concerns on this issue. Therefore, the outcome of current evidence strongly suggests that to assure optimal health and development, it is important to prevent and treat even mild ID of growing individuals, at least up to around 20 years of age, as well as during pregnancy. Over 200 million children worldwide do not reach their full

[4] Lúcia Helena Siva Miglioranza, PhD; Address: Department of Food Science and Technology. University of Londrina. Londrina, Paraná, Brazil. CEP: 86038-440. Telephone: (55) 43 33714984. E-mail: luciah@uel.br ; FAX: (55) 43 33714080.

[5] José Wander Breganó, PhD. Address: Department of Pathology, Clinical Analysis and Toxicology. Rua Robert Koch n° 60 Bairro Cervejaria, University of Londrina. Londrina, Paraná, Brazil. CEP: 86038-440. Telephone: (55) 43 3371 2200. E-mail: wbregano@onda.com.br. FAX: (55) 43 3371 2323

[6] Corresponding author: Isaias Dichi, MD, PhD. Address: Department of Internal Medicine. Rua Robert Koch n. 60 Bairro Cervejaria, University of Londrina. Londrina, Paraná, Brazil. CEP: 86038-440. Telephone: (55) 43 3371 2332. E-mail: dichi@sercomtel.com.br. FAX: (55) 43 3371 5100

development potential because of preventable causes, like iron deficiency. Fortification of food with iron, when an appropriate diet is not available, is considered the best sustainable way of preventing iron deficiency. The most difficult challenge to this end is to find the ideal combination of an iron fortified compound and its corresponding food vehicle. There exist many reports on the successful addition of sodium-iron ethylenediaminotetraacetate (NaFeEDTA) or ferrous bisglycinate fortifiers in the form of an iron chelate, which protects from combination with dietary inhibitors, mainly phytic acid. There is little evidence that iron fortification of staple foods, such as corn flour is a useful strategy to combat iron deficiency. However, some reports in Chile and Brazil seem to challenge this hypothesis. It could be argued that reports of marked decrease in iron absorption were verified with single meals, under special conditions, and that studies in which effects of enhancers and inhibitors of iron absorption were studied in whole meals showed results that were far less pronounced than those from single meals. Aside from these considerations, it should be emphasized that costs are very important in fortification measures, especially to convince political authorities in developing countries of the need for a continued Iron Fortification Program. Therefore, the aim of the present review is to study the different ways of fortification of food with iron in preventing and treating ID.

1. Introduction

All forms of malnutrition's broad spectrum are associated with significant morbidity, mortality, and economic costs, particularly in countries where both, under- and over nutrition co-exist, as is the case in developing countries undergoing rapid transition in nutrition and life-style [WHO, 2011].

Despite the great importance of the problems related to over nutrition, the consequences of under nutrition still remains spread worldwide, no matter if in developed or developing countries.

There are some highlights that deserve consideration in this approach. Iron deficiency (ID), for example, is the most common nutritional deficiency disorder in the world, affecting infants, children and women of childbearing age. In developing countries, every woman in the second pregnancy and about 40% of preschool children are estimated to be anemic, as consequence of ID.

ID occurs when the body is low in stored iron, it may not cause any symptoms and is often not recognized. In general, iron deficiency symptoms are considered to be due to an insufficient supply of iron to the tissues and probably not to lowered hemoglobin level. When it is detected, it can be treated with iron supplementation. If the low iron level or its cause is not corrected, it can lead to muscle weakness and eventually lead to iron deficiency anemia (IDA).

IDA is a condition that develops when a low iron level persists and prevents the body from making enough healthy red blood cells. The body can make red blood cells, even when it has an iron deficiency, but eventually the shortage of stored iron can slow that process and cause anemia.

The global prevalence of IDA for the general population is 24.8% and it is estimated that 1,6 to 2 billion people are affected by this disorder worldwide [World Health Organization, 2008]. It means that anemia affects one-quarter of the world's population and is concentrated in preschool-aged children and women, making it a global public health problem [Mc Lean, et al., 2009].

Although ID is responsible for at least half of the cases of anemia, there are other possible causes, including genetic, infectious, and other nutritional deficiencies. It is estimated that when anemia prevalence reaches 20%, ID exists in 50% of the population, and when anemia prevalence exceeds 40%, the entire population suffers from some degree of ID [Mc Lean et al., 2007].

The major health consequences from IDA are sub optimal pregnancy outcome including lower birth weight, increased morbidity in mothers and neonates, increased frequency and duration of upper respiratory infections in young children, delayed mental and motor development in young children with effects on behavior and cognitive performance when the child reaches school age, and reduced physical work capacity in adults.

It is currently known that, in many developing countries, iron deficiency anemia is frequently exacerbated by malaria and worm infections. ID is a problem even in developed countries such as the US, Canada and European countries.

The anemia estimates are provided by region for all population groups, based on data collected from 1993 to 2005 in the WHO Global Database on Anemia. The WHO Expert Consultation meeting, held in Geneva in 1992, defined the blood concentration of hemoglobin and established normal ranges for data assessment from different physiological groups of population, particularly children, adolescents, adults and pregnant women.

The numbers associated to the iron deficiency are impressive: in preschool-age children, the anemia prevalence is 47.4%, affecting 293 million children globally. The highest prevalence is in Africa (67.6%) and South-East Asia (65.5%). In the Eastern Mediterranean, the prevalence is 46% and around 20% in the other WHO regions: the Americas, Europe and Western Pacific.

For pregnant women the prevalence is slightly lower; however, its distribution by region follows the same trend as the one observed for preschool-age children. The highest prevalence is in Africa (57.1%) and in South-East Asia (48.2%), followed by the Eastern Mediterranean (44.2%), Western Pacific (30.7%), and the European and American regions, 25% and 24.1% respectively. Overall, 56.4 million pregnant women are anemic (41.8% prevalence globally).

In non-pregnant women, the prevalence of anemia is lower than in pregnant women. Overall, 468.4 million non-pregnant women are anemic (30.2% prevalence globally). The highest prevalence is found in Africa (47.5%) and in South-East Asia (35.7%). In the Eastern Mediterranean region, the prevalence is 32.4%, 20.5% in the Western Pacific region, 19% in the European region, and 17.8% in the Americas.

In sum, the global prevalence of anemia in school-age children is 25.4%, in men 12.7% and in elderly 23.9%.

All the numerical information was provided by compiled numbers of WHO, published in 2011. Despite the unfavorable numbers mentioned previously, the strategies used to fight against the present status are becoming more and more efficient, as verified with publications on iron fortification programs.

Low cost vehicles, extensive use of staple foods, biotechnology advances applied to the iron premix, and crops biofortification, are the proposed ways to change the status quo. And this is the focus of this chapter.

2. Consequences of Iron Deficiency in the Human Neurocognitive and Neurobehavioral Development

The human brain develops up until to about 20 years of age, and brain iron content also increases concomitantly up to this age. It may be difficult to repair negative effects of ID developed during this period.

During gestation, the fetus stores about 250 mg of iron. These stores are drawn on during breastfeeding, because breastmilk supplies only about 0.15 mg of absorbed iron per day, whereas requirements for absorbed iron are about 0.55 mg per day [Fomon, 1993]. Low birth weight infants do not store an adequate amount of iron during fetal life and are at high risk of developing iron deficiency while being breastfed. During growth in childhood, about 0.5 mg of iron per day is absorbed in excess of body losses; adequate amount of iron during growth typically results in a 70-kg man accumulating about 4 g of body iron [Institute of Medicine, 2001]. About 2.5 g of body iron is within hemoglobin and about 1 g is stored as ferritin or hemosiderin, mainly in the liver. An adult male absorbs and excrete about 0.8 mg of iron per day, and women, during childbearing years, should absorb almost twice as much (1.4 mg per day) to cover menstrual losses [Institute of Medicine, 2001].

Although there is a long way to elucidate all factors involved, the investigations into the role of iron in neurocognitive and neurobehavioral development are receiving much attention of researchers. The uptake of iron through the blood–brain barrier appears to be regulated and dependent on iron status [Beard, 2003]. Thus, there is a higher rate when iron status is low and a lower rate when it is high [Beard, 2003; Taylor et al., 1991]. In addition, this uptake process is highly selective and does not reflect overall blood–brain barrier permeability [Beard, 2003; Crowe and Morgan, 1992]. The brain obtains iron primarily via transferrin (Tf) and Tf receptors expressed in endothelial cells on the brain microvasculature [Beard, 2003, Han et al., 2003]. There appears to be a regulatory role for adjacent astrocytes in the regulation of this uptake across the blood–brain barrier [Osendarp, et al., 2010].

Following these assumptions, Badaracco et al. [2010] investigated oligodendrogenesis and myelination in rats at 3 days of age. It was verified that during early development ID causes specific changes in myelin composition, including a lower relative content of cholesterol, proteolipid protein (PLP), and myelin basic protein 21 (MBP21). The authors hypothesized that these changes could be a consequence of the adverse effects of ID on oligodendrocyte (OLGc) development and function, and their studies supports the concept that iron may affect OLGc development at early stages of embryogenesis rather than during late development. Also, observed that myelin composition is altered by a limited iron supply, changes that can be reverted by a single injection of apotransferrin (aTf).

Walker et al. [2007] reviewed biological and psychosocial risk factors that contribute to adverse outcomes and evaluated studies reporting poorer mental, motor, social-emotional, or neurophysiologic functioning in infants with iron deficiency anemia than those without, despite variation in study sample size and quality. All studies reported benefits of iron for motor outcomes, three reported social-emotional benefits, and cognitive-language benefits were seen in two studies. Those authors found only one systematic review that reported no effect of iron in infants, but there were several important parameters which were not considered in that study.

In reviewing the present literature, despite some inconclusive studies, the research results are pointing out to confirm that severe iron depletion during the neonatal period and infancy, causes a permanent deficit in cognitive, social and general life, achievements which lead to the conclusion that there is a critical period when a sufficient amount of iron is a prerequisite for basic brain developmental processes [Armano et al., 2010].

3. Old Strategies Results

The history of iron fortification is related in some ways to food fortification history. There are reports stating that food standards have existed since ancient Greece and Rome, however, as it is known today, dietary fortification of nutrients began in the 1920s. Previously, in 1831, the French physician Boussingault urged adding iodine to salt to prevent goiter. However, it was between the First and Second World Wars (1924-1944) that supplementation was established as a measure either to correct or prevent nutritional deficiencies in populations or to restore nutrients lost during food processing. Thus, at that time, it was established the adding of iodine to salt, vitamins A and D to margarine, vitamin D to milk, and vitamins B1, B2, niacin, and iron to flours and bread. Since the beginning, it was emphasized the health benefits accomplished through scientific research with the support of food manufacturers [Borenstein et al., 1971]. Therefore, since 1920, fortification has been a major strategy aimed at improving the nutritional quality of the food supply in industrialized countries for many decades but has only been applied in many developing countries recently.

Fortification of food with iron, when an appropriate diet is not available, is considered the best sustainable way of preventing iron deficiency. However, the challenge to reach this goal is to find the ideal combination of an iron fortified compound and its corresponding food vehicle. Many attempts to solve the problem have been investigated around the world and the staple food is the first strategy applied, to minimize rejection and intrinsic tendency to abandon the treatment in the public health level. In other words, the more widespread use of certain food (or vehicle) as iron carrier, greater is the chance of a successful intervention.

The effectiveness of iron fortification has been demonstrated in several world regions [WHO/FAO, 2006].

In Brazil, studies demonstrated the effectiveness of applying iron as ferrous sulphate at water, particularly for children from deprived areas, under social economics status of poverty [Dutra-de-Oliveira, et al., 1994; Beinner et al., 2005; Arcanjo et al., 2010]. Dutra-de-Oliveira et al. [1994] studies were conducted in day care centers and the results indicated that mean hemoglobin values increased from 10.6 to 13.7 g/dL and serum ferritin from 13.7 to 25.6 micrograms/L. Beinner et al. [2005] verified that daily consumption of iron-fortified drinking water in daycare facilities is an effective, simple and inexpensive way of reducing and controlling for moderate and severe anemia in pre-school children. The results of Arcanjo et al. [2010] pointed out greater adhesion and an increase in hemoglobin values, with a reduction in the prevalence of anemia with the consumption of drinking water fortified with 7.5 mg of elemental iron/L.

The Indian experience has been the use of common salt fortification successfully [Rao, 1994, Andersson et al., 2008; Shankar et al., 2009]. However, the prevalences of malaria, soil-transmitted helminths, and low intake of riboflavin as well as technological problems, did not allow that the same good results which were obtained in Ivory Coast, Africa [Wegmuller et al., 2006].

The Chinese government has started the project of promoting iron fortified soy sauce in some areas, covering a population of 60 million. Soy sauce was selected as the food carrier for a nation-wide iron fortification program in China sponsored by ILSI (International Life Science Institute) project IDEA (Iron Deficiency Eliminating Action) [Huo et al., 2007]. Despite the successful program, demonstrated by Chen in 2003, physicians in China raised concerns about the safety of the iron fortified compound, which was the sodium-iron ethylenediaminotetraacetate (NaFeEDTA). In 2006, the FDA assigned to NaFeEDTA the "Generally Recognized as Safe" (GRAS) status, through scientific procedures, for use as a source of dietary iron for fortification purposes in soy, plus teriyaki and hoisin (both soy based sauces), and fish sauces at a level of 0.024 percent iron by weight, and in sweet and sour sauce at a level of 0.012 percent iron by weight. Experts and researchers are optimistic about the results of this type of fortification in many studies worldwide [Bothwell et al., 2004; Van Thuy et al., 2005; Huo et al., 2007; Andersson et al., 2010].

Among attempts to choose the right staple foods, the most common are cereal based products. Worldwide, maize, rice and wheat flour are being fortified with ferrous sulfate, H-reduced iron or ferrous fumarate. The Sharing United States Technology to Aid in the Improvement of Nutrition [SUSTAIN, 2001] recommended preferably the use of ferrous sulfate, followed by ferrous fumarate and lastly electrolytic iron. In a recent review, Hurrel et al. [2010] evaluated iron fortification programs in 78 countries and verified that only nine national programs (Argentina, Chile, Egypt, Iran, Jordan, Lebanon, Syria, Turkmenistan, and Uruguay) had likely a significant positive impact on iron status of population. According those authors, most countries use non-recommended, low-bioavailability, atomized, reduced or hydrogen-reduced iron powders and as consequence, most current iron fortification programs are likely to be ineffective. Legislation needs updating in many countries to accomplish flour fortification with adequate levels of the recommended iron compounds.

Following the guidelines on food fortification [WHO/FAO, 2006], in order to ensure the successful fortification of wheat flour and wheat flour products, it may be necessary for individual countries to adopt different strategies taking into account differences in climate, wheat flour quality, processing methods and storage conditions, as well as differences in the main uses of flour (to make bread or other foods).

The importance of bread as a carrier for iron fortification may be verified in different cultures [Sadighi et al., 2008; Steyn et al., 2008; Vasconcelos et al., 2008]. Abu-Saad et al. [2010] evaluated the role of ethnic foods as predictors of intake levels of selected nutrients that are important during pregnancy among the Bedouin Arab minority population in southern Israel. The authors compared the main food predictors for Bedouin intakes of the selected nutrients with those for the Jewish majority population. They reported that homemade whole wheat bread was a main predictor of intake levels for five of the eight selected nutrients, and other ethnic foods/recipes, emerged as predictors of iron, folate, calcium, and n-3 fatty acid intakes. Fortification of cereal-grain products was introduced in 1941, when iron and three vitamins were added to flour and bread. Ready-to-eat cereals were fortified at about the same time. These fortifications have contributed to increased dietary iron intake and reductions in iron deficiency anemia in the United States [Whittaker et al., 2001].

Seal et al. [2008] investigated 157 children (6-59 months) from a population of Nangweshi refugee camp and anemia decreased by 23.4% associated with the introduction of maize meal fortification. Maize as carrier was also used in a study of Miglioranza et al. [2009] in Brazil, where the prevalence of ID and IDA among children and adolescents decreased from 18.0% and 14.9% to 5.6% and 1.2%, respectively, with ingestion of corn flour-derived products enriched with elemental Fe for six months. A survey carried out in Caracas in a population of 307 children aged 7, 11, and 15 y showed that the prevalence of iron deficiency determined by measuring the serum ferritin concentration were reduced from 37%, found in 1992, to 15%, found in 1994, as result of a fortification program with ferrous fumarate, in which precooked yellow and white maize were enriched with 20 mg Fe and wheat flours with 50 mg Fe/kg flour, respectively. These two cereals represent 45% of the total energy consumed daily by the low socioeconomic strata of the population [Layrisse et al., 1996]. Positive results were also found in South Africa, despite the lower bioavailability expected in iron fortified cereal studies. Faber et al. [2005] assessed whether fortified maize-meal porridge could reduce anemia and improve the micronutrient status and motor development of infants. The proportion of infants with anemia decreased from 45% to 17% in the fortified-porridge group, whereas it remained up to 40% in the control group. Hence, the authors emphasized the potential to reduce anemia with low-cost fortification.

In a study carried out by Andang´o et al. [2007] involving 516 children, aged 3-8 years in Kenya, they verified that consumption of maize flour with high-dose NaFeEDTA improved all measured iron-status indicators. Low-dose NaFeEDTA decreased the prevalence of iron deficiency but did not noticeably change the prevalence of anemia. Electrolytic iron did not improve any of these iron-status indicators. They pointed out that in high-phytate flours, NaFeEDTA is more suitable than electrolytic iron for supplementation of iron in the diet.

On the other hand, no matter if cereal or milk based foods, there are some concerns related to infant formulas. In 2003, Lynch and Stoltzfus suggested fortification levels for ferrous sulfate and ascorbic acid for some types of complementary foods targeted specifically for newborn infants until 24 months of age. They emphasized a need to develop formulas that ensure adequate dietary intake to meet specific requirements, since at that age ingested quantities may be quite small. They also warned that iron must be supplied in a highly bioavailable form. However, despite the high importance of an adequate iron intake by infants, few studies have reported iron fortification of baby food, and the available literature is almost limited to studies with infants at high nutritional risk [Moffatt et al., 1994]. Some authors even disapprove the fortification levels found in infant formulas prevailing in the food industry, arguing with the adverse effects that such products may cause [Moy, 2000], such as the interference with Cu and Se absorption or concerns about potential adverse effects on immune function and susceptibility to infections in gastrointestinal symptoms.

4. Promessing Strategies

Monotonous diet with low iron intake, and poor bioavailability is commonly mentioned as risk factors for iron deficiency [WHO/FAO, 2006]. Sensory limitations are presented in several fortified formulas. The already mentioned sodium-iron ethylenediaminotetraacetate (NaFeEDTA) or ferrous bisglycinate chelate have been recognized as successful fortifiers in diets which contain high levels of iron inhibitors, especially phytic acid. Those strategies could be particularly useful to enhance the bioavailability in staple foods around the world.

The necessity of viable fortification programs supports the persistence in staple foods inclusion, considering the premises that in developing countries, eating habits are strongly affected by their cost.

Wang et al. [2008] assessed the effect and safety of NaFeEDTA on Hb and serum ferritin in Fe-deficient populations. The authors performed a systematic review, identifying potential studies by searching the electronic databases of Medline, Cochrane Library, Embase, WHO Library and China National Knowledge Infrastructure. They concluded that NaFeEDTA increased both Hb and serum ferritin concentrations substantially in Fe-deficient populations, and could be the effective Fe preparation to combat Fe deficiency.

Positive performances were also found in investigations with iron chelate, as ferrous bisglycinate compound, despite its higher cost [Hertrampf et al., 2004; Van Stuijvenberg et al, 2006]. Amino acid chelates may be more useful in milk products and beverages [Hurrell et al, 2004] and there is a possibility of being used with inexpensive vehicles like whey beverages [Miglioranza et al, 2003] and cereal-based foods. Although bisglycinate is a more expensive source of iron than ferrous sulfate, smaller amounts could be used as a result of its higher bioavailability [Allen, 2002].

The concern of bioavailability has led scientists from *all* over the *world* to develop new products based on biotechnology, crops biofortification, encapsulation, and others (Table 1).

Similarly to China, India Biofortification Project has developed biofortified varieties of rice, as well as wheat, and maize. The biofortification strategy targets the undernourished by naturally adding nutrients to the staple foods through plant breeding [Tanumihardjo et al., 2008].

Dietary iron comprises non-heme (inorganic iron salts) and heme iron (animal origin), the latter being absorbed by a separate pathway and more efficiently than non-heme iron. The strategy adopted by some fortification programs includes using the heme-iron concentrated from animal origin, successfully applied to enhance bioavailability. Nakano et al, 2007, for example, studying rat diets, observed higher bioavailability in an iron-fortified whey protein concentrate (Fe-WPC) prepared by addition of ferric chloride compared to hemin that is an iron-containing porphyrin.

Microencapsulation technologies have also shown large applicability, particularly decreasing solubility problems, improving sensorial acceptance and increasing bioavailability. Encapsulated compounds also offer a possibility to fortify low-grade salt without causing off-colors or iodine loss [Hurrel, 2002].

The strategy using multiple micronutrients has been used in several countries [Chen et al., 2008; Ouedraogo et al., 2008; Tan et al., 2009; Osei et al., 2010; Sazawal et al., 2010] to improve iron intakes and, consequently, iron status, mostly for young children groups. In Mexico, Rosado et al. [2010] evaluated the efficacy of strategies that have recently been recommended to treat anemia. They applied an iron supplement, an iron+folic acid supplement, a multiple micronutrient supplement, a micronutrient-fortified complementary food as porridge powder, or zinc+iron+ascorbic acid fortified water, as treatment to 577 non-breastfed children, 6 to 43 mo of age.

Table 1. Some food choices and strategies for iron fortification, published between 2005 and 2010

Local	Food/ vehicle	Dietary strategy	Impact	Publication
China	Rice	Biofortification / higher nicotianamine concentration	Enhancement of bioavailability	Zheng et al., 2010
Canada	Iodized Salt	Encapsulated iron premix (ferrous fumarate)	Stability and iron bioavailability	Li et al., 2010
Mexico	Biscuits	Heme-iron concentrate from swine Hb	Enhancement of iron bioavailability	Gonzalez-Rosendo, et al., 2010
New Zealand	Milk Protein	Ferrous sulphate in protein iron complexes	Decreases solubility problems and the inhibition of lipid oxidation	Sugiarto et al, 2010
France	Casein micelles	Casein micelles loaded with ferric chloride	Creates a dispersible delivery format	Raouche et al., 2009
Vietnam	Biscuits	Multiple micronutrients (iron, zinc, iodine, vitamin A)	Reduction of anemia risk, enhanced deworming efficacy in schoolchildren	Tran et al., 2009
USA	Black beans	Biofortification	Increases iron intakes where beans is a dietary staple	Tako et al., 2009
India	Iodized Salt	Micronized ground ferric pyrophosphate and encapsulated ferrous fumarate	Both efficacious in reducing the prevalence of anemia and iron deficiency in school-age children	Andersson et al., 2008
Brazil	Rice	Ultra Rice technology: micronized ferric pyrophosphate (MPF)	Increased iron stores and reduced anemia in a group of mildly anemic children 6-24 mo old	Beinner et al., 2010
Kuwaiti	Wheat-based biscuits	Small particle-sized (40 μm) encapsulated FeSO4	Women aged 18-35 years, increased 88% body Fe stores	Biebinger et al., 2009

The conclusion of their studies was: the three supplements (iron, iron plus folic acid and iron plus micronutrients) increased Hb concentrations significantly more than fortified complementary food. According to the authors, the supplements that contained other micronutrients or folic acid were more effective for reducing the prevalence of anemia than fortified complementary food. In general, supplements were the least accepted among the food fortification strategies.

Rosado et al. [2010] also demonstrated that it is more important to consider other micronutrients than to provide high doses of iron alone. They emphasised that more attention should be given to other micronutrient deficiencies to increase the effectiveness of iron intervention programs.

Besides all those mentioned efforts, there is a key role for the food industry, in helping to improve habitual iron intakes and, more importantly, iron status with the use of scientific and technological applications. Derbyshire et al. [2010] remind some health improvements that may be associated with an increased use of functional foods. They warn, however, that fortified foods should be developed to reach all target groups and not just middle and high-income groups, populations who are not always at the greatest risk of micronutrient deficiencies.

Conclusion

Anemia affects one-quarter of the world's population and is concentrated mostly in infants, preschool-aged children and women of childbearing age, making it a global public health problem. It is becoming evident the importance of overcoming ID and IDA in early phases of life to avoid neurocognitive and neurobehavioral dysfunction. The ideal way to accomplish this objective would be through a nutritive diet. However, in developing countries where concerns about cost-effectiveness are always present, food fortification with iron remains a remarkable alternative.

NaFeEDTA seems to be the iron compound that better combines the fundamental duet effectiveness and cost. However, because of its good results, more studies with ferrous chelate bysblicinate are warranted, especially when milk is the vehicle. Staple food should be always considered as food vehicle since adding it to a habitual diet is an easy way to assure population adhesion. There are substantial reports of marked decrease in iron absorption verified with single meals, under special conditions. Also, there are enough studies in which effects of inhibitors of iron absorption were studied in whole meals showing results that were far less pronounced than those from single meals.

Many scientists agree that food fortification with iron should be part of a national priority policy and scientific communities, especially in developing countries, should make maximum efforts to convince political authorities of the need for a continued Iron Fortification Program.

References

Abu-Saad, K.; Shahar, D. R.; Vardi, H.; Fraser, D.(2010). Importance of ethnic foods as predictors of and contributors to nutrient intake levels in a minority population. *Eur J Clin Nutr*, 64,S88-S94.

Andang'o, P.E; Osendarp, S.J.; Ayah, R.; West, C.E.; Mwaniki, D.L.; De Wolf, C.A.; Kraaijenhagen, R.; Kok, F.J.; Verhoef, H. (2007). Efficacy of iron-fortified whole maize flour on iron status of schoolchildren in Kenya: a randomised controlled trial. *Lancet*, 369(9575), 1799-1806.

Andersson, M.; Thankachan, P.; Muthayya, S.; Goud, R. B.; Kurpad, A.V.; Hurrell, R. F.; Zimmermann, M. B.(2008). Dual fortification of salt with iodine and iron: a randomized, double-blind, controlled trial of micronized ferric pyrophosphate and encapsulated ferrous fumarate in southern India. *Am J Clin Nutr*, 88(5), 1378-1387.

Andersson, M.; Thankachan, P.; Muthayya, S.; Goud, R.B.; Kurpad, A.V.; Hurrell, R.F.; Zimmermann, M.B.(2008). Dual fortification of salt with iodine and iron: a randomized, double-blind, controlled trial of micronized ferric pyrophosphate and encapsulated ferrous fumarate in southern India. *Am J Clin Nutr*, 88(5):1378-1387.

Andersson, M.; Theis, W.; Zimmermann, M. B.; Foman, J. T.; J., Martín; D., Guus S. M. J. E.; Frenken, L. G. J.; Hurrell, R. F. (2010). Random serial sampling to evaluate efficacy of iron fortification a randomized controlled trial of margarine fortification with ferric pyrophosphate or sodium iron edetate. *Am J Clin Nutr*, 92(5), 1094-1104.

Arcanjo, F. P. N.; Arcanjo, C. C.; Amancio, O. M. S.; Braga, J. A. P.; Leite, A. J. M. (2011). Weekly Iron Supplementation for the Prevention of Anemia in Pre-school Children: A Randomized, Double-blind, Placebo-controlled Trial. *J Trop Pediatr* doi: 10.1093/tropej/fmq119

Armano, G.; Vulic, D.M.; Jovancevic, M. Konjarik, Z. (2010). Influence of iron deficiency on early brain development. *Paediatria Croatica*, 54(1), 47-52.

Badaracco, M.E.; Siri, M.V.; Pasquini, J.M. (2010). Oligodendrogenesis: the role of iron. *Biofactors*, 36 (2), 98-102.

Beard, J (2003). Iron deficiency alters brain development and functioning. *J Nutr*, 133 (Suppl), S1468–S1472.

Beinner, M. A.; Lamounier, J. A.; And Tomaz, C.(2005). Effect of Iron-Fortified Drinking Water of Daycare Facilities on the Hemoglobin Status of Young Children .*J Am Coll* Nutr, 24(2), 107-114.

Beinner, M. A.; Velasquez-Melendez, G.; Pessoa, M. C.; Greiner, T.(2010). Iron-Fortified Rice Is As Efficacious As Supplemental Iron Drops in Infants and Young Children. *J Nutr*, 140(1),49-53.

Biebinger, R.; Zimmermann, M.B.; Al-Hooti, S.N.; Al-Hamed, N.; Al-Salem, E.; Zafar, T.; Kabir, Y.; Al-Obaid, I.; Petry, N.; Hurrell, R.F. (2009). Efficacy of wheat-based biscuits fortified with microcapsules containing ferrous sulfate and potassium iodate or a new hydrogen-reduced elemental iron: a randomised, double-blind, controlled trial in Kuwaiti women. *Br J Nutr*, 102(9), 1362-1369.

Borenstein, B.; Lachance, P.(1971) Rationale and technology of food fortification with vitamins, minerals and aminoacids. *Critical Reviews in Food Science and Nutrition*, 2(2), 171 – 186.

Bothwell, T.H.; Macphail, A. P.(2004) .The potential role of NaFeEDTA as an iron fortificant. *Int J Vitam Nutr Res,* 74(6),421-34.

Chen, C. Iron fortification of soy sauce in China, 2003. Accessed at: ftp://ftp.fao.org/docrep/fao/005/y8346m/y8346m12.pdf, on february 04, 2011.

Chen, K.; Li, T.Y.; Chen, L.; Qu, P.; Liu, Y.X. (2008). Effects of Vitamin A, Vitamin A plus Iron and Multiple Micronutrient-Fortified Seasoning Powder on Preschool Children in a Suburb of Chongqing, China. *J Nutr Sci Vitaminol*, 54(6), 440-447.

Crowe, A.;_Morgan, E.H. (1992). Iron and transferrin uptake by brain and cerebrospinal fluid in the rat. Brain Res, 592,8-16.

Derbyshire, E.; Brennan, C. S.; Li, W.; Bokhari, F.(2010). Iron deficiency – is there a role for the food industry. *Int J Food Sci Tech*, 45: 2443–2448.

Dutra-de-Oliveira, J. E.; Ferreira, J. B.; Vasconcellos, V. P. Marchini, J.S.(1994). Drinking water as na iron carrier to control anemia in preschool children in a day-care center. *J Am Coll Nutr,* 13(2),198-202.

Faber, M.; Kvalsvig, J.D.; Lombard, C.J.; Benade, A.J.S. (2005). Effect of a fortified maize-meal porridge on anemia, micronutrient status, and motor development of infants. *Am J Clin Nutr*, 82(5), 1032-1039.

FDA Food and Drug Administration. GRAS Notice No. GRN 000178 CFSAN/Office of Food Additive Safety. January 11, 2006.

Fomon, S.(2001). Infant feeding in the 20th century: formula and beikost. *Journal of Nutrition*,131,409S-420S.

Fomon, S.J. (1993). Iron. In: Nutrition of Normal Infants. St. Louis: Mosby-Year Book, 239–59.

González-Rosendo, G.; Polo, J.; Rodríguez-Jerez, J.J.; Puga-Díaz, R.; Reyes-Navarrete, E.G.; Quintero-Gutiérrez, A.G.(2010). Bioavailability of a Heme-Iron Concentrate Product Added to Chocolate Biscuit Filling in Adolescent Girls Living in a Rural Area of Mexico. *J Food Sci*, 75(3), H73-H78.

Han, J.; Day, J.R.; Connor, J. R.; Beard, J. L.(2003) Gene expression of transferrin and transferrin receptor in brains of control vs. iron-deficient rats. *Nutr Neurosci*, 6,1-10.

Hertrampf, E.; Olivares, M. (2004). Iron amino acid chelates. *Int J Vitam Nutr Res*, 74(6), 435-443.

Huo, J.S.; Yang, X.G.; Piao, J.H.; Gao, J.Q.; Miao, H., Yu, B.; Lu, C. Q.; Chen, J.S.(2007). NaFeEDTA fortified soy sauce showed higher iron absorption rate in Chinese females. *Biomed Environ Sci*, 20(2),126-30.

Hurrel, R. F. (2002). Fortification: Overcoming technical and practical barriers. *J Nutr*, 132(4), 806S-812S.

Hurrell R, Ranum P, de Pee S, Biebinger R, Hulthen L, Johnson Q, Lynch S. (2010). Revised recommendations for iron fortification of wheat flour and an evaluation of the expected impact of current national wheat flour fortification programs. *Food Nutr Bull*, 31(1), S7-S21.

Hurrell, R. A. (1992). Prospects for improving the iron fortification of foods. In: Fomon, S. J.; Slotkin, S. eds. *Nutritional anemias*. New York: Raven Press.

Hurrell, R. A. (2004). Iron fortification: Current knowledge and promising new technologies. Flour Fortification Workshop: *Current Knowledge and Practical Applications* – Discussion Paper Cuernavaca, Mexico, 1-3.

Hurrell, R.F.; Lynch, S.; Bothwell, T.; Cori, H.; Glahn, R.; Hertrampf, E.; Kratky, Z.; Miller, D.; Rodenstein, M.; Streekstra, H.; Teucher, B.; Turner, E.; Yeung, C.K.; Zimmermann, M.B.(2004). Enhancing the absorption of fortification iron - A SUSTAIN Task Force report. *Int J Vitam Nutr*, 74(6), 387-401.

Institute Of Medicine (2001). Iron. In: Dietary Reference Intakes for Vitamin A, Vitamin K, Arsenic, Boron, Chromium, Copper, Iodine, Iron, Manganese, Molybdenum, Nickel, Silicon, Vanadium, and Zinc. Washington, DC: *National Academy Press*, 290-393.

Layrisse, M.; Chaves, J.F.; Bosch, V.; Tropper, E.; Bastardo,B.; Gonzalez, E. (1996). Early response to the effect of iron fortification in the Venezuelan population. *Am J Clin Nutr*, 64(6), 903-907.

Li, Y. O.; Diosady, L. L.; Wesley, A. S. (2010). Iodine stability in iodized salt dual fortified with microencapsulated ferrous fumarate made by an extrusion-based encapsulation process. *J Food Engin*, 99(2), 232-238.

Lynch, S.R.; Stoltzfus, R.J. (2003).Iron and ascorbic acid: Proposed fortification levels and recommended iron compounds. *J Nutr*,133(9), 2978S-2984S.

Mc Lean, E.; Egli, I.; De Benoist, B.; Wojdyla, D.; Cogswell, M. (2007). Worldwide prevalence of anemia in pre-school aged children, pregnant women and non-pregnant women of reproductive age. In: Kraemer, K., Zimmermann, M.B., eds. *Nutritional Anemia*. Basel, Switzerland: Sight and Life Press,1-12.

Mc Lean, E.; Cogswell, M.; Egli, I.; Wojdyla, D.; And De Benoist, B. (2009).Worldwide prevalence of anemia, WHO vitamin and mineral nutrition information system, 1993-2005. *Public Health Nutr*, 12, 444-454.

Miglioranza, L. H. S., Breganó, J. W., Dichi, I., Matsuo, T., Dichi, J. B., Barbosa, D. S.(2009). Effectiveness of fortification of corn flour-derived products with hydrogen-reduced elemental iron on iron-deficiency anaemia in children and adolescents in southern Brazil. *Public Health Nutr*, 12(2), 244-249.

Miglioranza, L.H.; Matsuo, T.; Caballero-Córdoba, G.M.; Dichi, J.B.; Cyrino, E.S.; Oliveira, I.B.; Martins, M.S.; Polezer, N.M.; Dichi, I.(2003). Effect of long-term fortification of whey drink with ferrous bisglycinate on anemia prevalence in children and adolescents from deprived areas of Londrina - PR, Brazil. *Nutrition*, 19(5), 419 – 421.

Moffatt, M.; Longstaffe, S.; Besant, J.;Ndureski, C. (1994). Prevention of iron-deficiency and psychomotor decline in high-risk infants through use of iron-fortified infant formula – a randomized clinical-trial. *J Pediatr*, 125(4), 527-534.

Moy, R.J.D.(2000). Iron fortification of infant formula. *Nutr Res Rev*, 13(2), 215-227, 2000.

Nakano, T.; Goto, T.; Nakaji, T.; Aoki, T. (2002). Bioavailability of iron-fortified whey protein concentrate in iron-deficient rats. *Asian Australas J Anim Sci*, 20 (7), 1120-1126.

OSEI, A. K.; ROSENBERG, I. H.; HOUSER, R. F.; BULUSU, S.; MATHEUS, M.; HAMER,D.H.(2010). Community-Level Micronutrient Fortification of School Lunch Meals Improved Vitamin A, Folate, and Iron Status of Schoolchildren in Himalayan Villages of India. *J Nutr*, 140(6),11-1154.

Osendarp, S. J.; Murray-Kolb, L. E; Black, M. M. (2010), Case study on iron in mental development – in memory of John Beard (1947–2009). Nutrition Reviews, 68, S48–S52.

Ouedraogo, H. Z.; Dramaix-Wilmet, M.; Zeba, A. N.; Hennart, P.; Donnen, P.(2008). Effect of iron or multiple micronutrient supplements on the prevalence of anaemia among anaemic young children of a malaria-endemic area: a randomized double-blind trial. *Trop Med Int Health*, 13(10), 1257-1266.

Rao, B.S.N. (1994). Fortification of salt with iron and iodine to control anaemia and goiter: Development of a new formula with good stability and bioavailability of iron and iodine. *Food Nutr Bull*,15,32-9.

Raouche, S.; Dobenesque, M.; Bot, A.; Lagaude, A.; Marchesseau, S. (2009).Casein micelles as a vehicle for iron fortification of foods. *Eur Food Res Tech*, 229(6), 929-935.

Rosado, J.L.; González, K.E.; Caamaño, M. del C.; García, O.P.; Preciado, R.; Odio, M. (2010). Efficacy of different strategies to treat anemia in children: a randomized clinical trial. *Nutrition J*, 9(40), 1-10.

Sadighi, J.; Sheikholeslam, R.; Mohammad, K.; Pouraram, H.; Abdollahi, Z.; Samadpour, K.; Kolahdooz, F.; Naghavi, M.(2008). Flour fortification with iron: a mid-term evaluation. *Public Health*, 122(3),313-321.

Sant, R. P.; Beverley, A. B.(2010). Undernutrition among children in South and South-East Asia. *J Paediatr Child Health*, 46(9), 497–503.

Sazawal, S.; Dhingra, U.; Dhingra, P.; Hiremath, G.; Sarkar, A.; Dutta, A.; Menon, V.P.; Black, R.E. (2010). Micronutrient Fortified Milk Improves Iron Status, Anemia and Growth among Children 1–4 Years: A Double Masked, Randomized, Controlled Trial. *PLoS ONE*, 5 (8), e12167.

Seal, A.; Kafwembe, E.; Kassim, I.A.; Hong, M.; Wesley, A.;Wood, J.; Abdalla, F.; van den Briel T. (2008). Maize meal fortification is associated with improved vitamin A and iron status in adolescents and reduced childhood anaemia in a food aid-dependent refugee population. *Public Health Nutr*, 11(7), 720-728.

Shankar, S.L.R.; Mathew, A.C.; Sivamani, M.; Banu, M.S.; Idupuganti, A.A. (2009). Fortification of salt with iodine and iron in India. *Am J Clin Nutr*, 90 (1), 246.

Steyn, N. P.; Wolmarans, P.; Nel, J. H.; Bourne, L. T. (2008). National fortification of staple foods can make a significant contribution to micronutrient intake of South African adults. *Public Health Nutr*, 11(3), 307-313.

Sugiarto, M.; Ye, A.; Taylor, M. W.; Singh, H. (2010). Milk protein-iron complexes: Inhibition of lipid oxidation in an emulsion. *Dairy Sci Technol*, 90(1), 87-98.

SUSTAIN Sharing United States Technology to Aid in the Improvement of Nutrition. Guidelines for Iron Fortification of Cereal Food Staples. Washington, DC, 2001.

Tako, E.; Laparra, J.M.; Glahn, R.P.; Welch, R..M.; Lei, X.G.; Beebe,D.; Miller, D.D. (2009). Biofortified Black Beans in a Maize and Bean Diet Provide More Bioavailable Iron to Piglets Than Standard Black Beans. *J Nutr*,139(2), 305-309.

Tanumihardjo, S.A.; Bouis, H.; Hotz, C.; Meenakshi, J.V.; McClafferty, B. (2008). Biofortification of staple crops: An emerging strategy to combat hidden hunger. *Comprehensive Reviews in Food Science and Food Safety*, 7(4), 329-334.

Taylor, E.M.;_Crowe, A.;_Morgan, E.H. (1991). Transferrin and iron uptake by the brain: effects of altered iron status. *J Neurochem*,57,1584-1592.

Tran, T. N.; Winichagoon, P.; Dijkhuizen, M. A.; Nguyen C. K.; Wasantwisut , E; Furr, H; Wieringa, F.T. (2009).Multi-Micronutrient-Fortified Biscuits Decreased Prevalence of Anemia and Improved Micronutrient Status and Effectiveness of Deworming in Rural Vietnamese School Children. *J Nutr*, 139(5), 1013-1021.

Van Stuijvenberg, M. E.; Smuts, C.M.; Wolmarans, P.; Lombard, C. J.; Dhansay, M. A.(2006). The efficacy of ferrous bisglycinate and electrolytic iron as fortificants in bread in iron-deficient school children. *Br J Nutr*, 95(3), 532-538.

Van Thuy P, Berger J, Nakanishi Y, Khan NC, Lynch S, Dixon P. (2005). The use of NaFeEDTA-fortified fish sauce is an effective tool for controlling iron deficiency in women of childbearing age in rural Vietnam. *J Nutr*, 135(11), 2596-601.

Vasconcelos, I. A. L.; Cortes, M. H.; Coitinho, D. C.(2008). Foods subject to mandatory fortification with iron: a study with pregnant women. *Rev Nutr*, 21(2), 149-160.

Walker, S. P.; Wachs, T.D.; Gardner, J. M.; Lozoff, B.; Wasserman, G. A. Pollitt, E. Carter, J. A. (2007). Child development: risk factors for adverse outcomes in developing countries. *Lancet*, 369(9556), 145-157.

Wang, B.; Zhan, S.; Xia, Y.; Lee, L.(2008). Effect of sodium iron ethylenediaminetetra-acetate (NaFeEDTA) on haemoglobin and serum ferritin in iron-deficient populations: a systematic review and meta-analysis of randomised and quasi-randomised controlled trials. *Br J Nutr*, 100(6), 1169-1178.

Wegmuller, R.; Camara, F.; Zimmermann, M. B.; Adou, P.; Hurrell, R. F. (2006). Salt Dual-Fortified with Iodine and Micronized Ground Ferric Pyrophosphate Affects Iron Status but Not Hemoglobin in Children in Cote *d'Ivoire*. *J Nutr,* 136(7), 1814-1820.

Whittaker, P.; Tufaro, P. R.; Rader, J.I. (2001). Iron and folate in fortified cereals. *J Am Coll Nutr*, 20(3), 247-254.

WHO World Health Organisation. Department of Nutrition for Health and Development. Captured on http://www.who.int/vmnis/anaemia/en/, january 31, 2011.

WHO World Health Organisation. Worldwide Prevalence of Anaemia 1993–2005: WHO Global Database on Anaemia. De Benoist, B.; Mc Lean, E.; Egli, I.; Cogswell, M. eds. Geneva, Switzerland: WHO Press, 2008.

WHO/ FAO. Diet, Nutrition and the Prevention of Chronic Diseases: report of a joint WHO/FAO expert consultation. WHO technical report series: 916. WHO; Geneva: 2003.

WHO/FAO. Guidelines on food fortification with micronutrients. ALLEN, LINDSAY et al. eds. WHO Press World Health Organization, 2006.

Yip, R.; Walsh, K.M.; Goldfarb, M.G.; Binkin N.J.(1987). Declining prevalence of anemia in childhood in a middle-class setting: a pediatric success story? *Pediatrics*, 80,330–334.

Zheng, L.; Cheng, Z.; Ai, C.; Jiang, X.; Bei, X.; Zheng, Y.; Glahn, R.P.; Welch, R.M.; Miller, D.D.; Lei, X.G.; Shou H. (2010). Nicotianamine, a Novel Enhancer of Rice Iron Bioavailability to Humans. *PLoS ONE*, 5(4), e10190.

In: Iron Deficiency and Its Complications
Editor: Yildiz Dincer
ISBN 978-1-61324-854-6

Chapter 6

Iron Deficiency Anemia in Pregnant Women

Andrew E. Czeizel[1*] *and Ferenc Bánhidy*[2]
[1]Foundation for the Community Control of Hereditary Diseases, Budapest, Hungary
[2]Second Department of Obstetrics and Gynecology, Semmelweis University, School of Medicine, Budapest, Hungary

Abstract

The aims of this research article are (i) to report new results of a population-based cohort study and (ii) to summarize the recent knowledge regarding the risk of iron deficiency anemia in pregnant women for adverse birth outcomes and the effective treatment of this pathological condition during pregnancy. The study design was the comparison the rate of preterm birth and low birthweight newborns of pregnant women with iron deficiency anemia according to the treatment of iron alone (N=1,576), iron + folic acid (N=4,419), folic acid alone (N=149) and without iron (and folic acid) treatment (N=214), in addition of pregnant women without iron deficiency anemia (N=31,793) as a reference group. Both iron deficiency anemia in pregnant women and the above adverse birth outcomes of newborns without birth defects were medically recorded in prenatal maternity logbook and discharge summary of women after delivery from inpatient obstetric clinics in the population-based Hungarian Case-Control Surveillance System of Congenital Abnormalities. There was a high rate of preterm births (15.0%) in the newborns of anemic pregnant women without iron treatment. The rate of preterm birth was only somewhat higher (10.7%) in the newborns of anemic pregnant women supplemented by iron compared to the figure of reference group (9.2%). However, anemic pregnant women with iron + folic acid treatment had a significantly lower rate of preterm

*Corresponding author: 1026 Budapest, Törökvész lejtő 32. Hungary. Tel/Fax 36 1 3944712, e-mail: czeizel@interware.hu

births (8.2%). The secondary findings of the study are the higher prevalence of constipation, hemorrhoids and hypotension in anemic pregnant women. These findings are discussed on the basis of data in the literature. In conclusion the higher risk of preterm birth of newborn infants born to pregnant women with iron deficiency anemia can be reduced by iron treatment and prevented by iron + folic acid supplementation.

Introduction

Anemia is defined as a hemoglobin value below the lower limits of normal range without the explanation of the dehydration state (Kilpatrick and Laros, 2004). However, anemia is not a disease but a sign similar to fever. The symptoms of anemia are caused by tissue hypoxia such as fatigue, lightheadedness, weakness and exertional dyspnoe. There are different causes of anemia; here the iron deficiency anemia is discussed because practically all persons with anemia belong to this group in Hungary.

The normal hemoglobin level is 14.0 ± 2.0 g/dL for adult female (Laros, 1986). Anemia is common in females because as the classical study of Scott and Pritchard (1967) showed the iron stores in healthy women are marginal at best due to the menstrual blood loss (25-30 ml containing 12-15 mg of element iron) in every female cycle.

The iron deficiency anemia is more common in pregnant women, thus if the previously mentioned definition of anemia is accepted, 20-60% of pregnant women will be found to be anemic at some time during the pregnancy (Alper et al., 2000).

Thus CDC defined anemia in pregnancy as a hemoglobin level below 11 g/dL in the first and third trimesters and below 10.5 g/dL in the second trimester (CDC, 1998). There are two different characteristics in pregnant women. On the one hand pregnancy is saved by 9 months of amenorrhea, i.e. blood loss.

On the other hand there is normally a 36% increase in the blood volume during pregnancy with a maximum at 34th gestation week (Peck and Arias, 1979). This drastic change is caused by the 47% plasma volume increase and 17 % red blood cell mass increase, the latter reaches its maximum at term. This difference results in a relative hemodilution throughout pregnancy with a maximum between 18 and 34 gestation weeks. However, the iron balance is a substantial demand for both pregnant women and the developing fetus, thus the usual diet in general cannot supply this large demand of iron, therefore supplementation of iron is necessary during pregnancy (Pritchard et al., 1969).

Previously the possible association of iron deficiency anemia in pregnant women with the risk of congenital abnormalities was evaluated without any higher risk (Bánhidy et al., 2010). The aim of this study was to check the possible association between iron deficiency anemia in pregnant women with or without iron treatment and the risk of their other adverse delivery/birth outcomes, particularly preterm birth and low birthweight newborns in the data set of the Hungarian Case-Control Surveillance of Congenital Abnormalities (HCCSCA) (Czeizel et al., 2001).

However, only the so-called controls, i.e. newborns without any defect are evaluated in the study because congenital abnormalities of cases may have a more robust effect for birth outcomes than iron deficiency anemia.

MATERIAL AND METHOD

The objective of the HCCSCA is to compare the exposures, e.g. maternal diseases, in the mothers of cases and controls during the study pregnancy.

Cases with different congenital abnormalities were selected from the Hungarian Congenital Abnormality Registry (Czeizel, 1997), while controls were identified in the National Birth Registry of the Central Statistical Office for the HCCSCA.

The definition of controls was newborn infants without any defect and in general two controls were matched with every case according to sex, birth week in the year when controls were born and district of parents' residence.

Data of exposures and confounders were collected from 3 sources:

1. Medically Recorded Prospective Data

Mothers of controls were asked in a mailed explanatory letter to send us the prenatal maternity logbook and other medical records (mainly discharge summaries of their deliveries) regarding their diseases and related treatments during the study pregnancy. Prenatal care was mandatory for pregnant women in Hungary (if somebody did not visit prenatal care, she did not get maternity grant and leave), thus nearly 100% of pregnant women visited prenatal care, on average seven times. The first visit was between 6th and 12th gestational weeks. Hemoglobin level, red blood cell count and hematocrit were measured in pregnant women at least during the first visit in the prenatal care clinic. The task of obstetricians was to record all pregnancy complications, maternal diseases and related drug prescriptions in the prenatal maternity logbook in the prenatal care clinics.

2. Retrospective Self-Reported Maternal Information

A structured questionnaire together with a list of diseases and drugs, and a printed informed consent were also mailed to the mothers immediately after the selection of controls. In order to standardise the answers, mothers were asked to read the enclosed list of diseases and medications as a memory aid before replying. Mothers were also asked to give a signature for informed consent which authorized us to record the name and address of their children in the HCCSCA.

The period between birth and return of "information package" (questionnaire, logbook, informed consent, etc.) in our prepaid envelop was 5.2 ± 2.9 months for controls.

3. Supplementary Data Collection

Our co-workers visited 200 non-respondent and 600 respondent control mothers as in the part of two validation studies (Czeizel et al., 2003, Czeizel and Vargha, 2004), as the ethic committee considered that this follow-up would be disturbing to all non-respondent mothers of healthy children. Our co-workers helped non-respondent mothers to fill-in the same questionnaire and to evaluate available medical documents. In addition our co-workers checked the previously reported data through a personal interview in respondent mothers. Finally they obtained data regarding lifestyle (smoking, drinking, and illicit drug use) during the study pregnancy through a personal interview of mothers and their close relatives living together in all the 800 mothers. The data of lifestyle were collected only in these subsamples due to the unreliability of retrospective maternal information (Czeizel et al., 2004).

Among potential *confounding factors,* maternal age, birth order, marital and employment status as indicator of socioeconomic status because it correlated well with the level of education and income, related drug treatments, and the use of pregnancy supplements were considered.

The available iron supplements included 50 (10 mg elementary Fe^{2+}), 70 and 100 mg ferrous sulfate in one tablet. In Hungary, only one kind of folic acid tablet was available during the study period and it contained 3 mg.

Finally necessary data were collected for 83.0% of controls (81.3% from reply, 1.7% from visit). The data of prenatal maternity logbooks were evaluated in these controls. Thus only prospectively and medically recorded diagnosis of iron deficiency anemia in the prenatal care logbook was evaluated in the study, because anemia reported retrospectively by mothers in the questionnaire frequently was not specified and/or without mentioning onset, duration, etc. Pregnancy complications were also evaluated on the medical record in the prenatal maternity logbook while the birth weight and gestational age at delivery were analyzed on the basis of discharge summary of deliveries. Gestational time was calculated from the first day of the last menstrual period. The rate of low birth weight (< 2500 g) and preterm births (< 37 weeks), in addition large birthweight (more than 4500 g) and postterm birth (over 42 weeks) were calculated. The diseases of mothers and related drugs treatments were evaluated on the basis of both medical records in the prenatal maternity logbook and the data of questionnaire filled-in by mothers. Finally the demographic data of mothers were analyzed on the basis of the questionnaire and discharge summary of deliveries.

The procedure of data collection was changed in 1997 because regional nurses visit and question all cases and controls, and the recent data had not been validated at the time of this analysis, thus only the data set of 17 years between 1980 and 1996 is evaluated here.

SAS version 8.02 (SAS Institute Inc., Cary, North Carolina, USA) was used for statistical analyses of data. At the evaluation of quantitative variables of birth outcomes (gestational age and birth weight) Student t test, while the evaluation of categorical birth outcomes such as preterm birth and low birthweight newborns odds ratio (OR) with 95% confidence interval (CI) were calculated. However, these risk figures were adjusted for maternal age, pregnancy order and socioeconomic status of mothers completed by gestational age in mean birth weight and the rate low birthweight newborns.

Results

Of 38,151 controls, i.e. newborns without any defect, 6,358 (16.7%) had mothers with medically recorded iron deficiency anemia in the prenatal maternity logbooks. Other types of anemia (in 2 pregnant women with hereditary spherocytosis) were excluded from the study.

Megaloblastic anemia was not recorded in the study sample of pregnant women. Thus the iron deficiency type of anemia will be mentioned later only as anemia.

The onset of anemia was recorded in the first gestational month in 688 (10.8%) mothers. The onset of their anemia was before the conception and continued during the study pregnancy, thus their anemia was considered as chronic. Thus anemia was diagnosed during the study pregnancy in about 90 % of pregnant women. The peak of new onset anemia was in the third gestational month (22.9%) explained by the laboratory examination of their blood at the first visit in the prenatal care clinics. This figure was 14.2% in mothers who visited the prenatal care clinic in the second gestational month. After the third gestational month there was a decreasing trend in the diagnosis of anemia: 17.5% in the fourth, 12.1% in the fifth, 9.0% in the sixth and 7.6% in the seventh gestational months of pregnant women. Later the diagnosis of anemia was rare. The question is whether these pregnant women had a true new onset anemia or their anemia was only diagnosed in these gestational months.

Of 6,358 pregnant women with anemia, 1,576 (24.8%) were treated with iron, while 4,419 (69.5%) had iron + folic acid treatment. However, 214 (3.4%) pregnant women with anemia were not treated with iron (and folic acid) and 149 (2.3%) had only folic acid treatment. The main objective of this study is to compare the birth outcomes of newborn infants born to the above pregnant women and compared to the reference group including 31,793 pregnant women without anemia. However, 65.3 % of pregnant women without anemia had iron supplementation and 51.0 % of them used of folic acid for the prevention of neural-tube defects.

The main characteristics of mothers in different study groups are shown in Table 1. The mean maternal age was somewhat lower due to the higher proportion of young age group (19 yr or less) in pregnant women with anemia except in the group without iron treatment. The mean birth order did not show obvious difference among the study groups. The mean birth order (birth + miscarriages) was the same in all but one study group, and the exception was again pregnant women without iron supplementation. This 0.3 difference instead of the other 0.2 difference may indicate a somewhat higher rate of miscarriages in previous pregnancies. The proportion of unmarried status was not significantly different among the study groups. However, the distribution of maternal employment status as indicator of socioeconomic status is worth mentioning. The proportion of high educated professional pregnant women was the larger in the groups of females without iron treatment and iron + folic acid supplementation. The latter is understandable because this combined treatment seems to be more effective during pregnancy. However, the high proportion of professional females among pregnant women without iron treatment needs some explanation. Some of these females wanted to have "natural" pregnancy without any artificial effect, including iron supplementation.

In the subsample of 800 control mothers visited at home, 114 (14.5%) were recorded as anemic and 15 (12.9%) smoked during the study pregnancy, while of 684 control mothers without anemia, 137 (20.0%) had smoking habit during the study pregnancy. The drinking habit was also evaluated but the rate of hard/regular drinkers was about 1 % in all subsamples. The incidences of acute maternal disease groups (including at least 5 pregnant women in the reference group) are shown in Table 2. The incidence of some acute disease groups such as influenza-common cold (particularly the latter with secondary complications), urinary tract and genital organs was higher in pregnant women with anemia compared to pregnant women without anemia.

Table 1. Main variables of mothers in the different study groups

Variables	Reference group (N=31,793)		Iron supplement-ation (N=1,576)		Iron+folic acid supplement-ation (N=4,419)		Folic acid supplement-ation (N=149)		No treatment (N=214)	
Quantitative	No.	%	No.	%	No.	%	No.	%	No.	%
Maternal age (yr) -19 or less	2,669	8.4	165	10.5	397	9.0	24	16.1	22	10.3
20-29	22,976	72.3	1,134	72.0	3,235	73.2	109	73.2	148	69.2
30 or more	6,148	19.3	277	17.6	787	17.8	16	10.7	44	20.6
Mean±S. D.	25.5	4.9	25.1	4.8	25.3	4.7	24.5	4.7	25.6	5.1
Birth order 1	15,131	47.6	726	46.1	2,164	49.0	78	52.3	110	51.4
2 or more	16,662	52.4	850	53.9	2,255	51.0	71	47.7	104	48.6
Mean S.D.	1.7	0.9	1.8	0.9	1.7	0.9	1.7	1.2	1.8	1.1
Pregnancy order 1	13,549	42.6	673	42.7	1,927	43.6	74	49.7	97	45.3
2 or more	18,244	57.4	903	57.3	2,492	56.4	75	50.3	117	54.7
Mean S.D.	1.9	1.2	1.9	1.1	1.9	1.1	1.9	1.2	2.1	1.5
Categorical	*No.*	*%*	*No*	*%*	*No.*	*%*	*No.*	*%*	*No.*	*%*
Unmarried	1,245	3.9	56	3.6	161	3.6	4	2.7	6	2.8
Enployment status professional	3,641	11.5	165	10.5	577	13.1	11	7.4	29	13.6
managerial	8,511	26.8	404	25.6	1,262	28.6	32	21.5	56	26.2
skilled worker	10,058	31.6	485	30.8	1,251	28.3	52	34.9	62	29.0
semiskilled worker	5,020	15.8	312	19.8	771	17.4	28	18.8	30	14.0
unskilled worker	1,837	5.8	95	6.0	228	5.2	12	8.1	15	7.0
housewife	1,976	6.2	96	6.1	256	5.8	7	4.7	19	8.9
Others	750	2.4	19	1.2	74	1.7	7	4.7	3	1.4

Table 2. Incidence of acute maternal disease groups in different study groups

Acute disease groups	Reference group (N=31,793)		Iron supplementation (N=1,576)		Iron+folic acid supplementation (N=4,419)		Folic acid (N=149)		No treatment (N=214)	
	No.	%	No.	%	No.	%	No.	%	No.	%
Influenza, common cold	5,917	18.6	369	23.4	880	19.9	30	20.1	65	30.4
Influenza	1,483	4.7	78	4.9	208	4.7	8	5.4	14	6.5
Common cold with secondary complications	4,434	13.9	291	18.5	672	15.2	22	14.8	51	23.8
Respiratory system	3,209	10.1	144	9.1	439	9.9	21	14.1	34	15.9
Upper part	2,707	8.5	117	7.4	394	8.9	20	13.4	28	13.1
Lower part	502	1.6	27	1.7	45	1.0	1	0.7	6	2.8
Digestive system	677	2.1	22	1.4	99	2.2	4	2.7	4	1.9
Diarrhoae	82	0.3	3	0.2	8	0.2	0	0.0	0	0.0
Orofacial herpes	476	1.5	12	0.8	78	1.8	2	1.3	3	1.4
Viral hepatitis	13	0.0	1	0.1	1	0.0	0	0.0	1	0.5
Gastritis and duodenitis	61	0.2	6	0.4	9	0.2	2	1.3	0	0.0
Others	5	0.0	0	0.0	1	0.0	0	0.0	0	0.0
Urinary tract	1,861	5.9	130	8.2	311	7.0	7	4.7	19	8.9
Upper part	309	1.0	19	1.2	54	1.2	1	0.7	6	2.8
Lower part	1,552	4.9	111	7.0	257	5.8	6	4.9	13	6.1
Genital organs	2,368	7.4	162	10.3	376	8.5	16	10.7	15	7.0
Vulvovaginitis	2,218	7.0	153	9.7	355	8.0	16	10.7	9	4.2
Pelvic inflammatory disease	103	0.3	6	0.4	12	0.3	0	0.0	6	2.8
Genital herpes	18	0.1	1	0.1	5	0.1	0	0.0	0	0.0
Viral warts	20	0.1	2	0.1	3	0.1	0	0.0	0	0.0
Other genital infections	2	0.0	0	0.0	0	0.0	0	0.0	0	0.0
Rest of disease	373	1.2	14	0.9	42	1.0	1	0.7	1	0.5
Other infections disease	66	0.2	1	0.1	6	0.1	0	0.0	1	0.5

Table 2. (Continued)

Acute disease groups	Reference group (N=31,793)		Iron supplementation (N=1,576)		Iron+folic acid supplementation (N=4,419)		Folic acid (N=149)		No treatment (N=214)	
	No.	%	No.	%	No.	%	No.	%	No.	%
Otitis media	49	0.2	2	0.1	4	0.1	0	0.0	0	0.0
Rubella	27	0.1	2	0.1	8	0.2	1	0.7	0	0.0
Mumps	37	0.1	2	0.1	10	0.2	0	0.0	0	0.0
Dermatomycosis	64	0.2	4	0.3	3	0.1	0	0.0	0	0.0
Ascariasis	7	0.0	1	0.1	2	0.0	0	0.0	0	0.0
Toxoplasmosis	25	0.1	1	0.1	1	0.0	0	0.0	0	0.0
Cytomegalic inclusion disease	45	0.1	1	0.1	3	0.1	0	0.0	0	0.0
Others	5	0.0	0	0.0	1	0.0	0	0.0	0	0.0

In addition anemic pregnant women without iron treatment had a very high incidence of common cold and acute diseases of respiratory system and urinary tract.

Among chronic diseases (Table 3), three showed some general association with maternal anemia. There was a high prevalence of constipation in general started after the onset of iron supplementation. The higher prevalence of constipation may explain the higher prevalence of hemorrhoids, frequently bleeding in our pregnant women, and this pathological condition certainly had a role in the origin of maternal anemia. The higher prevalence of hypotension in anemic pregnant women is noteworthy. On the other hand anemic pregnant women without iron treatment show a different pattern - beyond the previously mentioned 3 pathological conditions with the highest prevalence – because there were 7 diabetic pregnant women (3.3%) among them, in addition 5 (2.3%) had affective (depression or maniac-depressive) disorders, while 19 (11.7%) were affected with essential hypertension and 14 (6.5%) had thrombophlebitis. Thus these pregnant women can be classified as a high risk group.

The incidence of medically recorded pregnancy complications was also evaluated in mothers with anemia compared to mothers without anemia (Table 4). In fact the incidence of threatened abortion and severe treated nausea-vomiting was higher in all study groups of anemic pregnant women. However, the highest incidence of severe nausea-vomiting occurred in anemic pregnant women without iron (and folic acid) treatment, thus this association may be connected mainly with anemia and not with anemia related treatment. Gestational hypertension was recorded also more frequently in anemic pregnant women without iron treatment. There was no significant difference in the distribution and frequency of other drug uses between anemic pregnant women with or without different treatment and the reference group, i.e. pregnant women without anemia.

The main objective of the study was the evaluation of birth outcomes of newborn infants in the different study groups (Table 5). There was no difference in the sex ratio and twin rate among the study groups. The mean gestational age at delivery was the same in the newborns of anemic pregnant women with folic acid use (39.4 wk) than in the reference group. However, there were small differences in the groups of iron treatment (39.3 wk) and iron + folic acid use (39.5 wk) compared to the reference group, but these differences are not important from clinical aspect. However, there was 0.5 week shorter mean gestational age in 214 anemic pregnant women without iron supplementation ($t=2.2$; $p=0.03$).

These data were in the agreement with the rate of preterm birth. This rate was very high in Hungary during the study period and the figure of reference group (9.2%) reflected it. Anemia is a risk factor in the origin of preterm birth because its rate was 15.0% in the newborns of anemic pregnant women without iron (and folic acid) treatment (OR with 95% CI: 1.67, 1.11-2.10). The iron supplementation alone was not able to reduce this risk because the rate of preterm birth was higher in the group of anemic pregnant with iron treatment (10.7%) and nearly the same in the group of folic acid (9.4%). However, iron + folic together were able to reduce the rate of preterm birth to 8.2%, near to the level of significance (OR with 95% CI: 0.87, 0.67-1.08). The mean birth weight was only 8 g smaller in the group of anemic pregnant women with iron treatment than in the reference group. However, this difference was minus 41 g between the reference group and anemic pregnant women without iron (and folic acid) treatment ($t=0.1$; $p=0.91$). On the other hand anemic pregnant women had 73 g larger mean birth weight after folic acid treatment, though iron + folic acid treatment resulted in only 7 g plus.

Table 3. Prevalence of medically recorded chronic maternal diseases in different study groups

Chronic disease	Reference group (N=31,793)		Iron supplementation (N=1,576)		Iron+folic acid supplementation (N=4,419)		Folic acid supplementation (N=149)		No treatment (N=214)	
	No.	%	No.	%	No.	%	No.	%	No.	%
Diabetes nellitus	205	0.6	4	0.3	13	0.3	0	0.0	7	3.3
Epilepsy	84	0.3	1	0.1	5	0.1	0	0.0	0	0.0
Thyroid disorders	114	0.4	7	0.4	15	0.3	3	2.0	3	1.4
Psychiatric disease	161	0.5	12	0.8	30	0.7	2	1.3	5	2.3
Affective disorders	156	0.5	12	0.8	29	0.7	2	1.3	5	2.3
Others	5	0.0	0	0.0.	1	0.0	0	0.0	0	0.0
Neurological disease	600	1.9	32	2.0	82	1.9	4	2.7	7	3.3
Migraine	590	1.9	32	2.0	75	1.7	4	2.7	7	3.3
Others	10	0.0	0	0.0	7	0.2	0	0.0	0	0.0
Cardiovascular disease	4,818	15.2	313	19.9	957	21.7	28	18.8	80	37.4
Essential hypertension	1,394	4.4	45	2.9	132	3.0	2	1.3	19	8.9
Thrombophlebitis, embolism	725	2.3	56	3.6	178	4.0	5	3.4	14	6.5
Conduction disorders	122	0.4	9	0.6	20	0.5	0	0.0	5	2.3
Haemorrhoids	1,222	3.8	91	5.8	278	6.3	8	5.4	25	11.7
Varicose veins of lower extremities	445	1.4	34	2.2	82	1.9	3	2.0	2	0.9
Hypotension	899	2.8	76	4.8	265	6.0	10	6.7	15	7.0
Others	11	0.0	2	0.1	2	0.0	0	0.0	0	0.0
Respiratory system	424	1.3	9	0.6	70	1.6	3	2.0	3	1.4
Allergic rhinitis/asthma	404	1.3	9	0.6	68	1.5	3	2.0	2	0.9
Others	20	0.1	0	0.0	2	0.0	0	0.0	1	0.5
Digestive system	1,028	3.2	86	5.5	251	5.7	6	4.0	27	12.6
Dyspepsia/reflux	120	0.4	2	0.1	12	0.3	0	0.0	1	0.5
Colitis	80	0.3	10	0.6	7	0.2	1	0.7	3	1.4
Constipation	530	1.7	60	3.8	190	4.3	2	1.3	17	7.9

Chronic disease	Reference group (N=31,793)		Iron supplementation (N=1,576)		Iron+folic acid supplementation (N=4,419)		Folic acid supplementation (N=149)		No treatment (N=214)	
	No.	%	No.	%	No.	%	No.	%	No.	%
Cholacystis, cholelithiasis	225	0.7	9	0.6	29	0.7	2	1.3	4	1.9
Others	73	0.2	5	0.3	13	0.3	1	0.7	2	0.9
Urinary tract	123	0.4	9	0.6	12	0.3	1	0.7	5	2.3
Nephrolithiasis	123	0.4	8	0.5	12	0.3	1	0.7	5	2.3
Others	0	0.0	1	0.1	0	0.0	0	0.0	0	0.0
Genital organs*	185	0.6	9	0.6	25	0.6	0	0.0	4	1.9
Skin	135	0.4	4	0.3	16	0.4	1	0.7	3	1.4
Adverse allergic drug reaction	148	0.5	8	0.5	29	0.7	0	0.0	2	0.9
Skeletal system	151	0.5	11	0.7	27	0.6	1	0.7	3	1.4
Congenital abnormalities	123	0.4	5	0.3	25	0.6	1	0.7	1	0.5
Others**	51	0.2	3	0.2	2	0.0	0	0.0	0	0.0

*ovarian cyst, leiomyoma, etc.

**neoplasm, endocrine, etc.

Table 4. Incidence of medically recorded pregnancy complications in the different study groups

Pregnancy complications	Reference group (N=31,793)		Iron supplementation (N=1,576)		Iron+folic acid supplementation (N=4,419)		Folic acid supplementation (N=149)		No treatment (N=214)	
	No.	%	No.	%	No.	%	No.	%	No.	%
Threatened abortion	5,284	16.6	287	18.2	869	19.7	32	21.5	38	17.8
Nausea-vomiting, severe	3,041	9.6	184	11.7	582	13.2	18	12.1	31	14.5
Pre-eclampsia	945	3.0	46	2.9	150	3.4	7	4.7	8	3.7
Gestational hypertension	914	2.9	46	2.9	119	2.7	6	4.0	15	7.0
Pregnancy related renal diseases	383	1.2	33	2.1	71	1.6	1	0.7	4	1.9
Edema-excessive weight gain*	669	2.1	68	4.3	163	3.7	5	3.4	7	3.3
Gestational diabetes	199	0.6	7	0.4	21	0.5	0	0.0	2	0.9
Placental disorders**	500	1.6	15	1.0	74	1.7	1	0.7	3	1.4
Polyhydramnios	146	0.5	10	0.6	31	0.7	0	0.0	4	1.9
Oligohydramnios	13	0.0	0	0.0	1	0.0	0	0.0	0	0.0
Threatened preterm delivery***	4,378	13.8	221	14.0	802	18.1	18	12.1	28	13.1
Prolonged pregnancy	378	1.2	31	2.0	90	2.0	2	1.3	4	1.9
Others****	128	0.4	11	0.7	30	0.7	0	0.0	1	0.5

*without hypertension.

**incl. placenta previa, premature separation of placenta and antepartum hemorrhage.

***incl. cervical incompetence as well.

****e.g. trauma, poisoning, blood isoimmunisation, etc.

Table 5. Birth outcomes of newborn infants born to iron deficiency anemic pregnant women with different treatments and without treatment, in addition pregnant women without anemia as reference group

Variables	Reference group (N=31,793)		Iron supplementation (N=1,576)		Iron+folic acid supplementation (N=4,419)		Folic acid supplementation (N=149)		No treatment (N=214)	
Categorical	No.	%	No.	%	No.	%	No.	%	No.	%
Preterm birth	2,9191	9.2	168	10.7	363	8.2	14	9.4	32	15.0
Postterm birth	553	1.7	33	2.1	94	2.1	2	1.3	3	1.4
Low birthweight	1,850	5.8	70	4.4	226	5.1	5	3.4	16	7.5
Large birthweight	2,416	7.6	95	6.0	332	7.5	15	10.1	14	6.5
Quantitative	*Mean*	*S.D.*	*Mean*	*S.D*	*Mean*	*S.D.*	*Mean*	*S.D.*	*Mean*	*S.D.*
Gestational age (wk)	39.4	2.1	39.3	2.1	39.5	2.0	39.4	2.0	38.9	2.3
Birthweight (g)	3,275	513	3,267	482	3,282	505	3,348	470	3,234	545

The rate of low birthweight newborns was 5.8 % in the reference group, and this rate was higher (7.5%) but not significantly in untreated anemic pregnant women (OR with 95% CI: 1.37, 0.75-2.19). (The lack of significance is explained mainly by the limited number of pregnant women.) Iron, iron + folic acid and particularly folic acid treatment reduced this risk in the newborns of anemic pregnant women.

There was no significant difference in the rate of postterm birth and large birthweight newborns among the study groups.

Discussion

The efficacy of iron supplementation during pregnancy in anemic pregnant women was studied on the basis of adverse birth outcomes of their newborn infants.

Iron deficiency anemia associated with a somewhat higher risk of preterm birth after iron supplementation birth. However, the newborns of pregnant women with early diagnosis of anemia but without iron treatment had a significantly shorter gestational age at delivery and much a higher rate of preterm births. However, this risk can be neutralized by iron + folic acid supplementation.

Iron deficiency anemia did not associate with a higher risk of low birthweight newborns after iron supplementation. However, a significantly higher rate of low birthweight was found in the newborns of anemic pregnant women without iron (and folic acid) supplementation. Folic acid may have a more obvious effect for birth weight and the rate of low birthweight newborns than iron. In conclusion our study indicated a significantly higher rate of adverse birth outcomes of anemic pregnant women without iron treatment. Iron treatment was appropriate to reduce the rate of low birthweight newborns of anemic pregnant women, but the combined use iron + folic acid supplementation seems to be optimal in iron deficiency anemia of pregnant women.

Previous studies showed a higher risk of preterm birth and low birthweight newborns (Klebanoff et al., 1991, Lu et al., 1991, Scholl et al., 1992, Goldenberg et al., 1996), in addition of stillbirth (Sagen et al., 1984, Stephansson et al., 2000) of anemic pregnant women. However, recent studies including a meta-analysis of available data, reported only a significant association between anemia in early pregnancy and higher risk of preterm birth (Scanlon et al., 2000, Xiong et al., 2000, Bondevik et al., 2001). The higher risk of preterm delivery/birth in pregnant women with anemia during the first and second trimesters was explained by three hypotheses: (i) Hypoxia in the placenta and fetus. (ii) Increased oxidative stress in iron-deficient women cannot be neutralized by endogenous or dietary antioxidants. (iii) Reduced immune function due to iron deficiency associates with a higher risk of infection with increased production of inflammatory cytokines, secretion of corticotropin-releasing hormone and production of prostaglandin (Allen, 2001). The higher risk of some infectious/inflammatory diseases of anemic pregnant women was confirmed in this study as well. However, the main message of our study is that iron deficiency anemia does not pose a risk for pregnant women and their fetuses if pregnant women are treated appropriately. Recent meta-analyses of available data also showed that mild and/or treated iron deficiency anemia may associate with little harm to either pregnant women or the fetus (Scholl and

Hediger, 1994, Xiong et al., 2000, Kilpatrick and Laros, 2004). However, Cochrane database analyses suggested "further studies are needed to asses the effects of routine antenatal supplementation with iron or a combination of iron and folic acid on clinically important maternal and infant outcomes (Pena-Rosas and Viteri, 2006, 2009). Our hope is that our contribution may help to asses better the complications of anemic pregnant women and it is worth combining the effect of iron and folic acid, because our recent study showed that folic acid in the third trimester of pregnancy can reduce the rate of preterm birth (Czeizel et al., 2010).

The secondary finding of the study was an association of anemia with constipation and constipation related hemorrhoids. The cause of the so-called new-onset "pregnancy constipation" mainly in the third and fourth gestational months is connected with the common oral iron therapy during pregnancy which may exacerbate constipation (Williamson 2001, Welsh 2004, Ács et al., 2010). This observation can be explained by the well-known secondary relation between constipation and hemorrhoids, frequently bleeding in our pregnant (Bánhidy et al., 2010a). However, our data are against the statement that iron treatment is the main cause of nausea-vomiting in pregnant women (Gill et al., 2009). Finally our findings showed an association of anemia with hypotension (Bánhidy et al., 2010b), the question is whether these pathological conditions have common or independent origin.

Anemic pregnant women without iron (and folic acid) treatment showed a higher incidence of some acute diseases such as common cold with secondary complications and a higher prevalence of some chronic diseases such as essential hypertension. However, the limited number of these pregnant women avoided a detailed analysis of their data.

The prevalence of iron deficiency anemia during the study pregnancy was 16.7% in pregnant. This fact is explained by the "dilution" role of pregnancy in the origin of anemia, i.e. expansion of the plasma volume and the increasing demand of iron during pregnancy. Thus the usual diet in general cannot supply this large demand on iron, therefore supplementation of iron is necessary during pregnancy.

In conclusion our study showed that iron deficiency anemia with iron and particularly iron + folic acid supplementation does not pose a risk of adverse birth outcomes for pregnant women and their fetuses. Thus iron and folic acid supplementation results in a significant benefit for anemic pregnant women.

References

Ács N, Bánhidy F, Puho HE, Czeizel AE: No association between severe constipation with related drug treatment in pregnant women and congenital abnormalities in their offspring - a population-based case-control study. *Congenit Anom*. 2010;

Allen LH. Anemia and iron deficiency: Effects on pregnancy outcomes. *Am J Clin Nutr*. 2000; 71: 1280S-1284S.

Alper BS, Kimber R, Reddy AK: Using ferritin levels to determine iron deficiency anemia in pregnancy. *J Fam Pract*. 2000; 49: 829-833.

Bánhidy F, Ács N, Puho HE, Czeizel AE: Iron deficiency anemia: Pregnancy outcomes with or without iron supplementation. *Nutrition*, 2009; 12: 005/ 2010 Apr 7.

Bánhidy F, Ács N, Puho HE, Czeizel AE: Possible association of maternal haemorrhoid with congenital abnormalities in their children - a population-based case-control study. *Balkan J Med Genet.* 2010a; 13: 23-33.

Bánhidy F, Ács N, Puho HE, Czeizel AE: Hypotension in pregnant women: - a population-based case-control study of pregnancy complications and birth outcomes. *Hypertens Res.* 2010b; doi: 10.1038/hr.2010.172.

Bondevik GT, Lie RT, Ulstein M et al: Maternal hematological status and risk of low birth weight and preterm delivery in Nepal. *Acta Obstet Gynaecol Scand.* 2001; 80: 1402-1410.

CDC: Centers for Disease Control and Prevention: Recommendation to prevent and control iron deficiency anemia in the Unites States MMWR (Morb Mortal Wkly Rep) 1988; 47: 1-16.

Czeizel AE. The first 25 years of the Hungarian Congenital Abnormality Registry. *Teratology*, 1997; 55: 299-305.

Czeizel AE, Vargha P. Periconceptional folic acid/multivitamin supplementation and twin pregnancy. *Am J Obstet Gynecol.* 2004; 191: 790-794.

Czeizel AE, Rockenbauer M, Siffel Cs, Varga E. Description and mission evaluation of the Hungarian Case-Control Surveillance of Congenital Abnormalities, 1980 -1996. *Teratology*, 2001; 63: 176-185.

Czeizel AE, Petik D, Vargha P. Validation studies of drug exposures in pregnant women. Pharmacoepidemiology *Drug Safety*, 2003; 12: 409-416.

Czeizel AE, Petik D, Puho AE. Smoking and alcohol drinking during pregnancy. The reliability of retrospective maternal self-reported information. *Cent Eur J Publ Health*, 2004; 12: 179-183.

Czeizel AE, Puho HE, Langmar Z, et al. Possible association of folic acid supplementation during pregnancy with reduction of preterm birth: a population-based study. *Eur J Obstet Gynecol Reprod Biol.* 2010; 148: 135-140.

Gill SK, Maltepe G. Koren G. The effectiveness of discontinuing iron-containing prenatal multivitamins on reducing the severity of nausea and vomiting of pregnancy. *J Obstet Gynecol.* 2009; 29: 13-16.

Goldenberg RJ, Tamura T, DuBard M et al: Plasma ferritin and pregnancy outcome. *Am J Obstet Gynecol.* 1996; 175: 1356-1362.

Kilpatrick SJ, Laros RK: Maternal hematologic disorders. In: Creasy RK, Resnik R, Iams JD (eds.): Maternal-Fetal Medicine. 5th ed, Saunders, Philadelphia, 2004. pp. 975-1004.

Klebanoff MA, Shiono PH, Shelby JV et al: Anemia and spontaneous preterm birth. *Am J Obstet Gynecol.* 1991; 59: 164-169.

Laros RK Jr. (ed.): Blood Disorders in Pregnancy. Lea and Febiger, Philadelphia, 1986.

Lu ZM, Goldenberg RL, Cliver SP et al: The relationship between maternal hematocrit and pregnancy outcomes. *Obstet Gynecol.* 1991; 77: 190-195.

Peck TM, Arias F: Hematologic changes associated with pregnancy. *Clin Obstet.* 1979; 22: 785-791.

Pena-Rosas JP, Viteri FE. Effects of routine oral iron supplementation with or without folic acid for women during pregnancy. *Cochrane Database Syst Rev.* 2006; 19(3): CD004736.

Pena-Rosas JP, Viteri FE. Effects and safety of preventive oral iron or iron+folic acid supplementation for women during pregnancy. *Cochrane Database Syst Rev*. 2009; 7(4): CD004736.

Pritchard JA, Whalley PJ, Scott DE: The influence of maternal folate and iron deficiency on intrauterine life. *Am J Obstet Gynecol*. 1969; 104: 388-393.

Sagen N, Nilsen ST, Kim HC et al: Maternal hemoglobin concentration is closely related to birth weight in normal pregnancy. *Acta Obstet Gynaecol Scand*. 1984; 63: 245-256.

Scanlon KS, Yip R, Schieve LA, Cogswell ME: High and low hemoglobin levels during pregnancy. Differential risks for preterm birth and small for gestational age. *Obstet Gynecol*. 2000; 96: 741-747.

Scholl TO, Hediger ML, Fischer RL et al: Anemia vs. iron deficiency: Increased risk of preterm delivery in a prospective study. *Am J Clin Nutr*. 1992; 55: 985-991.

Scott DE, Pritchard JA: Iron deficiency in healthy young college women. *JAMA* (J Am Med Ass) 1967; 199: 147-153.

Stephansson O, Dickman PW, Johansson A et al: Maternal hemoglobin concentration during pregnancy and risk of stillbirth. *JAMA* (J Am Med Ass) 2000, 284: 2611-2618.

Welsh A. Hyperemesis, gastrointestinal and liver disorders in pregnancy. *Curr Obstet Gynaecol*. 2005; 15: 123-131.

Williamson C. Gastrointestinal disease. *Best Pract Res Clin Obstet and Gynaecol*. 2001; 15: (No. 5) 937-952.

Xiong X, Buekens P, Alexander S et al: Anemia during pregnancy and birth outcomes: a meta-analysis. *Am J Perinatol*. 2000; 17: 137-142.

In: Iron Deficiency and Its Complications
Editor: Yildiz Dincer
ISBN 978-1-61324-854-6

Chapter 7

Iron Deficiency Anemia and Its Complications

Modisa S. Motswaledi * ***and Ishmael Kasvosve***
Department of Medical Laboratory Sciences,
Faculty of Medicine and Health Sciences,
University of Botswana, Gaborone, Botswana

Abstract

Iron deficiency is a common nutritional disorder worldwide and it is estimated that 841 000 deaths occur annually due to iron deficiency or its complication. The common causes of iron deficiency are increased demand in pregnant and growing children, poor dietary intake, and increased blood losses due to parasitic infections and disorders such as malignancy and gastrointestinal bleeding. This review article discusses the clinical and laboratory diagnosis of iron deficiency. Iron–deficient erythropoiesis will be discussed along with the key biochemical markers of iron depletion and homeostasis. The role of iron in various catalytic and selected biochemical pathways will be discussed. Storage of iron in the reticulo-endothelial system and derangements in the biochemical pathways for regulation of ferrokinetics will be discussed with emphasis on the role of membrane proteins (transferrin-transferrin receptor, hepcidin, ferroportin, etc) as well as how specific cytokines such as IL-6, TNF-α, etc, contribute to iron homeostasis.

The review will also discuss the complications of iron deficiency, particularly those associated with cardiovascular, immunological and neurological disorders. The paper will discuss longitudinal studies both in humans and animal models to demonstrate neural mal-developments and long term effects of iron deficiency, including psychomotor, cognitive and affective derangements. The cardiovascular discussion of the complications of IDA will include a pathophysiological treatment of hypoxia as it affects the development of cardiomyopathy, cardiac insufficiency, hypoperfusion and angina. The

* Corresponding author: Department of Medical Laboratory Sciences, Faculty of Medicine and Health Sciences, University of Botswana. Private Bag 712, Gaborone, Botswana. Email: modisa.motswaledi@mopipi.ub.bw

risk of thrombosis associated with IDA will be discussed with particular reference to stroke occurring in children and infants. The review will also discuss the role of iron deficiency in the regulation of the immune system. In particular, the effect of iron deficiency on the production of cell-mediated and humoral immune responses and how such factors as cytokines and other products of the immune system affect the metabolism of iron will be discussed.

INTRODUCTION

Iron deficiency is a common nutritional disorder worldwide occasioning over 800,000 deaths annually with as much as 71% of its deaths and disabilities being borne by Africa and Asia alone (Stoltzfus, 2003), (Gillespie, 1991). It is most common among women of childbearing age and growing children due to increased physiological demands. IDA may also occur due to low dietary iron intake or increased blood loss as a result of parasitic infections chronic hemolysis or disorders such as malignancies that lead to gastrointestinal bleeding (Brittenham, 2009) or parasitic infections. In pregnancy, anemia may be aggravated by the dilutional effect of fluid retention (ReedGroup, 2011). In infants, the increased demand to support growth may be further aggravated by poor dietary iron intake, especially where milk is the sole or major diet (Finnegan, 2009).

Iron is essential for life and is required for numerous biochemical reactions in the body. Cytochromes are a group of iron-containing enzymes that are required for electron transport chain in the mitochondria in the production of ATP (Galan, 1984). Other enzymes such as catalase and peroxidase which are needed for detoxifying hydrogen peroxide generated in various biochemical reactions also contain iron. Myeloperoxidase and lactoferrin are important for bactericidal activity of polymorphonuclear leukocytes (Bullen, 1981), (Hill, 2004) while ribonucleic reductase is needed for DNA synthesis. Tyrosine hydroxylase, another iron-containing enzyme is responsible for dopamine synthesis in brain cells (Hoffmann, 2003). All these are examples of iron-containing enzymes whose function can be severely impaired by a deficiency of iron. Iron is also required for the synthesis of hemoglobin and myoglobin. Hemoglobin is essential to life as it transports oxygen to all parts of the body. It follows then that the pathology of iron deficiency would be manifested in processes that involve these enzymes. Indeed deficiencies have been observed in energy production, phagocytic activity, neural development and immune cell proliferation in iron deficiency.

IRON ABSORPTION AND KINETICS

The most common biological form of iron is the ferric (Fe^{3+}) (Goswami, 2002), in which form it exists in food, in circulation bound to transferrin and in storage form as ferritin (Zhang, 2009). The ferric (Fe^{3+}) rather than the ferrous (Fe^{2+}) is implicit in the naming of these iron-binding molecules. Iron must be reduced to the ferrous form in order to render it more soluble and biologically active. In the intestinal lumen, this is achieved through the action of the duodenal cytochrome B (DCytB) reductase. This conversion enables it to be absorbed via the divalent metal transporter 1 (DMT1) into the enterocyte *en route* to the basolateral surface where it is exported into the plasma through the universal iron exporter, ferroportin (Zhang, 2009). In the process of exportation into plasma, Fe^{2+} is converted back to Fe^{3+} by the action of hephaestin, a trans-membrane protein closely associated with ferroportin (Yeh, 2009). Ferroportin is also responsible for mobilizing iron from storage cells (enterocytes, macrophages and hepatocytes) into circulation. A genetic defect in the ferroportin molecule results in hemochromatosis, a pathological accumulation of iron in storage cells (Pietrangelo, 2004).

Transferrin is an iron-binding glycoprotein that serves as the main currency for exchange of plasma iron at cellular level (Goswami, 2002). A single molecule of transferrin can bind up to two molecules of iron. The concentration of transferrin effectively represents the iron-binding capacity. When iron is abundant in the body, such as in hemolytic anemias, transferrin is relatively saturated with iron while a deficiency of iron is reflected by low transferrin saturation. True iron deficiency results in increase in transferrin levels along with cell-membrane transferrin receptors (TfR), which are required for binding and internalizing the transferrin-bound iron. TfR is expressed on the cell membranes of all cells, including iron-storage cells (Salmon, 1985). In iron deficiency anemia, some of the transferrin receptors are shed in plasma as soluble transferrin receptors (sTfR) and can be used as a marker of true iron deficiency anemia as compared to anemia of chronic disease (Gupta, 2009).

Role of Hepcidin in Iron Homeostasis and Anemia of Inflammation

The availability of iron in circulation reflects the balance between ferroportin and a hepatocyte-derived circulating protein, hepcidin. Hepcidin derives its name from its source as well as its antibacterial and antifungal effects (Park, 2001). It binds ferroportin on the cell membranes and causes its internalization and degradation. This diminishes the number of iron-exporting molecules from the storage cells and thus reduces plasma iron (Weiss, 2005) while increasing iron stores. In chronic infections, sustained levels of inflammatory cytokines are responsible for elevated levels of hepcidin. Hepcidin also reduces intestinal absorption of iron (Rossi, 2005). Hepcidin is therefore considered the basic biochemical explanation of iron sequestration in the face of severe need in anemia of chronic disorders (ACD) (Inamura, 2005). The depletion of circulating iron by hepcidin levels is thought to be a coordinated defense mechanism designed to deprive bacteria of the iron needed for their biochemical reactions (Bullen, 1981).

As an acute phase reactant, hepcidin production is stimulated by the presence of bacterial lipopolysaccharides as well as by other inflammatory cytokines such as IL-6 (Rossi, 2005), (Weiss, 2005). Evidence of increased protein synthesis in any cell can be demonstrated by the increase in the number of specific mRNAs for that protein. On the basis of this concept, in vitro experiments using human hepatocytes have demonstrated that hepcidin mRNA synthesis is stimulated by administration of IL-6 and IL-1β (Inamura, 2005), while Nemeth et al concluded that IL-6 is the "necessary and sufficient cytokine for the induction of hepcidin during inflammation" (Nemeth, 2004).

A study by Yanoff and colleagues revealed similar findings that higher levels of inflammatory indicators were associated with anemia of chronic disorders in obese subjects

(Yanoff, 2007). Furthermore, Bekri et al observed that hepcidin is also produced in adipocytes of severely obese subjects (Bekri, 2006). Therefore the anemia of obesity may represent true IDA or anemia similar to that of chronic inflammation. Prolonged inflammation as occurs in chronic disease therefore tends to maintain the body in a state of chronic iron deprivation through heightened hepcidin levels, ultimately leading to anemia of chronic disorders, also termed anemia of inflammation. Chronic inflammation is therefore a cause rather than a complication of this type of iron deficiency.

In the absence of infection, however, plasma hepcidin levels are responsive to cellular oxygen needs, being decreased under anemic or hypoxic conditions (Zhang, 2009), where erythropoiesis necessitates iron mobilization from storage cells. Thus, hepcidin is considered the most important regulator of plasma iron levels (Rossi, 2005).

Diagnosis of Iron Deficiency Anemia

Iron deficiency does not necessarily result in anemia (Jan, 2003). However, where the severity is sufficient to manifest as anemia, patients may present with easy fatigability and pallor. Other clinical observations may include angular cheilitis, spooning of the nails and glossitis (Brittenham, 2009). Loss of hair is becoming increasingly recognized as a complication of iron deficiency anemia and has been associated with decreased serum ferritin levels (Rushton, 2003), (Kantor, 2003).

Laboratory findings include a microcytic hypochromic anemia commonly accompanied by thrombocytosis. The reticulocyte count is characteristically low or normal unless the patient has recently commenced some form of treatment. Iron deficient erythropoiesis results in erythroid hyperplasia with small normoblasts showing a ragged cytoplasm (Finnegan, 2009). Plasma transferrin levels are high with an increased expression of transferrin receptors (Khumalo, 1988). Iron stores in the bone marrow and reticuloendothelial system are characteristically depleted as are those of plasma ferritin. The anemia develops when the iron stores are depleted and is initially normochromic with anisocytosis before the hypochromia develops (College of Physicians and Surgeons of Alberta, 2008).

Free erythrocyte propotoporphyrin is another test for iron deficiency. Under normal circumstances, iron is incorporated into the protoporphyrin ring to form heme by the action of the enzyme ferrochelatase in the synthesis of hemoglobin. In the absence of iron, however, zinc is incorporated leading to formation of zinc protoporhyrin (ZPP), or free erythrocyte protopophyrin (FEP). FEP can therefore be used to confirm the diagnosis of IDA, although it may also be elevated in other conditions such as lead poisoning.

Complications of Iron Deficiency

Cardiovascular Complications

Severe iron deficiency anemia can cause cardiovascular complications. Iron deficiency anemia may result in reduced amount of oxygen supply to body organs and myocardium and consequently, a higher volume of blood is required to supply the same amount of oxygen.

Cardiac output is thus increased in compensatory response which may lead to cardiac enlargement and reduction of ventricular volume. The resulting cardiac hypoperfusion may result in cardiac arrhythmia and angina. This may ultimately result in cardiac failure with symptoms such as edema of the legs and the lungs. Furthermore, this hypoperfusion may lead to fetal loss or preterm delivery in pregnant women (Huang, 2010).

Iron deficiency is commonly accompanied by thrombocytosis. Although thrombocytosis is generally not considered a risk factor for thrombosis (Schafer, 2004), (Hartfield, 1997), there is increasing evidence implicating iron deficiency in thrombotic events. Both carotid artery and cerebral venous thromboses have been reported as possible sequelae to IDA with or without thrombocytosis (Akins, 1996). Kinoshita et al describe two cases in which cerebral venous thrombosis occurred in adults in whom IDA was the only identifiable pathology (Kinoshita, 2006). Since these patients had normal platelet counts, it can be concluded that other factors than thrombocytosis contribute to thrombosis in iron deficiency anemia. In fact, Sébire et al observed that high levels of Factor VIII and homozygosity for methylene tetrahydrofolate reductase polymorphism were additional risk factors in children (Sébire, 2005) while Hartfield et al related the thrombosis in their patients to a viral prodrome (Hartfield, 1997). Other risk factors include the severity of the anemia and hypercholesterolemia (Stolz, 2007). Whatever the cause, IDA appears to promote an environment conducive for thrombus formation by various triggers. The role of iron deficiency in thrombotic disorders is reviewed more extensively by Franchini et al (Franchini, 2008)

Incidences of stroke in children are comparatively rare, (Yager, 2008), (Belman, 1990). However, the incident of stroke occurring in children with iron deficiency anemia warrants special attention due to the growing number of reported cases, often in association with other conditions but also in those patients where iron deficiency is the only pathology identifiable (Franchini, 2008), (Yager, 2008). Characteristically, the patients appear to be infants or children under the age of five years with the risk increasing with age (Yager, 2008). In one case a 27-month-old baby suffered a cerebral infarction with IDA being the only preceding condition (Ready, 1989). Other cases involved a child with concomitant kidney disease but again with thrombocytosis and anemia (Meena, 2000), a case of stroke occurring in six children aged six to eighteen months with IDA and thrombocytosis (Hartfield, 1997), and a 22-month old infant with cerebral venous thrombosis, IDA and thrombocytosis (Belman, 1990). In childhood, therefore, IDA-related strokes do occur with sufficient frequency to warrant attention.

Neurological Complications

The role of iron deficiency in the development of the brain is well documented (Beard, 2003). Children born to iron-deficient mothers have been shown to have increased risk of preterm delivery as well as delayed neurological development (King, 2006). Longitudinal studies (pre-school to adolescence) of iron deficient children have demonstrated long-term suboptimal development of cognitive, motor and socio-emotional capacities (Lozoff, 2006) persisting well into adolescence (Madan, 2010), (Lukowski, 2010). These studies made the striking observation that a student's IQ at later years of development can be predicted by various measures of iron such as hemoglobin, ferritin, etc at earlier stages of development.

These defects were attributable to deranged neural development and function as a consequence of IDA. Iron deficiency interferes with normal development of neuronal networks and myelination of nerve fibres. Further evidence suggests that the neuronal and myelination maldevelopments are irreversible and target specific regions of the brain resulting in aberrations of dopamine receptors and transporters (Beard, 2003). A study of school children with Attention Deficit Hyperactivity Disorder (ADHD) who were referred for school problems in France found that the level of iron in the form of ferritin was approximately half of those in the control group. These results corroborate the evidence that iron is necessary for dopamine synthesis, a stimulant that is deficient in ADHD patients. The severity of ADHD was correlated with levels of ferritin (Kennedy M. , 2005).

Iron Deficiency and Immunity

Iron deficiency diminishes lymphocyte DNA synthesis, proliferation and function (Brock, 2000). Lymphocyte proliferation involves synthesis of DNA, for which Fe^{2+} is required. Lederman et al demonstrated that removal of iron using deferoxamine actually inhibits the incorporation of radio-labeled thymidine into new DNA thereby preventing its synthesis and cell proliferation. This inhibition was completely reversed by removal of deferoxamine or addition of stoichiometric amounts of Fe^{3+} (Lederman, 1984).

Moreover, a study of IDA patients by Santos and Falcão documented significantly lower CD3, CD4 and B cell counts as well as diminished lymphocyte cytotoxicity in IDA patients compared to controls. These deficiencies were corrected after the patients received iron treatment (Santos, 1990). Subsequent studies by other investigators corroborated these findings. For example, Mullick et al found lower T-lymphocyte counts, including CD4+ cells in IDA along with a lower CD4:CD8 ratio (Mullick, 2006). This reversed CD4:CD8 ratio favors T-suppressor over T-helper function and therefore compromises overall immunity. Iron deficient T-cells are also less responsive to *in vitro* activation as shown by diminished proliferation (Ahluwalia, 2004). Ekiz et al reported IDA patients to have significantly lower levels of Interleukin-6 (IL-6) compared to controls as well as low levels of IgG4 (Ekiz, 2005), evidence that supports the role of iron deficiency in curtailing B- and T-lymphocyte functions.

The inhibition of tumor necrosis factor alpha (TNF-α) production has been demonstrated in iron-deficient subjects (Lopez, 2003). It remains to be confirmed whether this is a normal and desired adaptation to anemia since the presence of TNF-α would aggravate anemia by promoting iron storage rather than its mobilization, as well as by inhibiting erythropoiesis (Weiss, 2005). In any case, the overall impact of this lack of TNF-α most likely contributes to the susceptibility of iron-deficient subjects to infection, especially in the light of other suppressed immune functions described above.

Iron deficiency has also been shown to inhibit the phagocytic and bactericidal activity of neutrophils and macrophages. This is consistent with the well-established role of lactoferrin and myeloperoxidase, iron-binding or containing proteins found in neutrophils (Bullen, 1981). Other investigations found that IDA polymorphonuclear phagocytes (neutrophils) showed less phagocytic activity than controls, and that their phagocytic activity was restored by addition of iron (Bergman, 2005). However, higher doses of iron resulted in diminished phagocytic activity and may explain the aggravation of infection in one study involving IDA patients (Murray, 1978). Murray et al observed an increased activation of latent infections in Somali subjects following iron supplementation and proposed that iron deficiency in these subjects was protective. Therefore, a balance appears to be necessary between the need to deprive the invading microorganisms of iron and the need to provide for the body's own biochemical needs, including the oxidative burst necessary for microbicidal activity.

Conclusion

Iron is needed for normal function by various body organs. It is required for hemoglobin synthesis and oxygen transport to all tissues. Iron is a component of many enzymes that are crucial for normal cell function. Plasma iron concentrations are controlled by hepcidin and are inversely related to those of hepcidin. Hepcidin production increases in response to inflammation and inhibits the mobilization of intracellular iron by binding ferroportin and inducing its internalization and subsequent degradation. It also inhibits intestinal absorption of iron and suppresses erythropoiesis. Inflammatory conditions that increase hepcidin secretion therefore reduce circulating iron and provide explanation for the mechanism of anemia of chronic inflammation.

Iron deficiency anemia places a strain on cardiac function and may lead to cardiac failure and death. IDA is also implicated in promoting a thrombotic environment as seen by the occurrence of stroke in iron-deficient adults and infants.

Iron deficiency impairs proliferation and activity of lymphocytes as well as the phagocytic and respiratory burst responsible for bactericidal activity of neutrophils. Cytokine production is inhibited as are levels of some antibodies.

Iron is important for brain development. Iron deficient infants have brain developmental deficits involving poor neuronal development, defective development of dopamine and dopamine receptors with consequent cognitive and psychosocial maldevelopments.

References

Ahluwalia, N. S. (2004). Immune function is impaired in iron-deficient, homebound, older women. *Am J Clin Nutr* , *79*, 516-21.

Akins, P. G. (1996). Carotid Artery Thrombus Associated With Severe Iron-Deficiency Anemia and Thrombocytosis. *Stroke* , *27*, 1002-1005.

Alberta, College of Physicians and Surgeons of. (2008, March). *Hematology Morphology Critique*. Retrieved March Thursday, 2011, from Alberta Laboratory Quality Enhancement Program: http://www.cpsa.ab.ca/Libraries/Pro_QofC_ALQEP_ Critiques/Critique_08-03-S.pdf

Beard, J. (2003). Iron Deficiency alters brain development and functioning. *J. Nutr* , *5 Suppl 1*, 1468S-72S.

Bekri, S. G. (2006). Increased Adipose Tissue Expression of Hepcidin in Severe Obesity Is Independent From Diabetes and NASH. *GASTROENTEROLOGY* , *131*, 788–796.

Belman, A. R. (1990). Cerebral Venous Thrombosis in a Child With Iron Deficiency Anemia and Thrombocytosis. *Stroke , 21* (3), 488-493.

Bergman, M. S. (2005). Phagocytic capacity and apoptosis of peripheral blood cells from patients with iron deficiency anemia. *Biomedicine and Pharmacotherapy , 59*, 307-11.

Brittenham, G. (2009). Disorders of iron metabolism: iron deficiency and iron overload. In R. B. Hoffman, *Hematology: Basic Principles and Practice* (pp. 453-468). Philadelphia: Churchill Livingstone Elsevier.

Brock, J. M. (2000). Cellular and molecualr aspects of iron and immune function. *Proc Nutr Soc , 59*, 537-540.

Bullen, J. (1981). The significance of iron in infection. *Rev Infect Dis. , 3* (6), 1127-28.

Ekiz, C. A. (2005). The effect of iron deficiency anemia on the function of the immune system. *The Hematology Journal , 5*, 579–583.

Finnegan, K. (2009). Iron Metabolism and Hypochromic Anemias. In D. Harmening, *Clinical Hematology and Fundamentals of Hemostasis* (5 ed., pp. 117-137). Philadelphia: F. A. Davis.

Franchini, M. T. (2008). Iron and thrombosis. *Ann Hematol , 87* (3), 167-173.

Galan, P. H. (1984). The activity of tissue enzymes in iron-deficient rat and man: an overview. *Comp Biochem Physiol B , 77* (4), 647-5.

Ganz, T. (2003). Hepcidin a key regulator of iron metabolism and mediator of anemia of inflammation. *Blood , 102* (3), 783-788.

Gillespie, S. M. (1991). *Controlling iron deficiency - State-of-the-art series nutrition policy discussion paper no. 9.* Geneva: Gillespie S, Mason JB, Kevany J, eds. ControlliUnited Nations Administrative Committee on Coordination/Subcommittee on Nutrition.

Goswami, T. R. (2002). Iron transport: emerging roles in health and disease. *Biochem. Cell Biol. , 80*, 679-689.

Gupta, S. U. (2009). Is soluble transferrin receptor a good marker of iron deficiency anemia in chronic kidney disease patients? *Indian J Nephrol , 19* (3), 96–100.

Hartfield, D. L. (1997). Iron deficiency: a cause of stroke in infants and children. *Pediatr Neurol. , 16* (1), 50-3.

Hill, H. B. (2004). The Natural (innate) Defense System. In E. O. Steihm, *Immunological Disorders in Infants and Children* (pp. 245-269). Philadelphia: Elsevier Saunders.

Hoffmann, G. A.-V.-S. (2003). Tyrosine hydroxylase deficiency causes progressive encephalopathy and dopa-nonresponsive dystonia. *Ann Neurol , 54* (Suppl 6), S56-65.

Huang, S. Y. (2010). The etiology and treatment outcome of iron deficiency and iron deficiency anemia in children. *J Pediatr Hematol Oncol. , 32* (4), 282-5.

Inamura, J. I. (2005). Upregulation of hepcidin by interleukin-1beta in human hepatoma cell lines. *Hepatol Res. 2005 Nov;33(3):. Epub 2005 Sep 29. , 33* (3), 198-205.

Jan, A. M. (2003). Non-anemic iron deficiency - Diagnostic perspective. *JK-Practitioner , 10* (1), 47-48.

Kantor, J. K. (2003). Decreased Serum Ferritin is AssociatedWith Alopecia inWomen. *J Inves Dermatol , 121* (5), 985-988.

Kennedy, M. (2005). ADHD and iron Deficiency Anemia: Are they linked? *American Journal of Nursing , 105* (3), 22-22.

Khumalo, H. G. (1988). Serum transferrin receptors are decreased in the presence of iron overload. *Clinical Chemistry* , 40-44.

King, D. (2006). Iron Deficiency. *Journal of Childbirth Education* , 32(4).

Kinoshita, Y. T. (2006). Cerebral venous thrombosis associated with iron deficiency anemia. *Neurol Med Chir(Tokyo)* , *46*, 589-593.

Lederman, H. C. (1984). Deferoxamine: A reversible S-phase inhibitor of S human lymphocyte proliferation. *Blood* , *64* (3), 748-753.

Lopez, M. R. (2003). Tumour necrosis factor-α transcription in transferrin-stimulated human blood mononuclear cells: is transferrin receptor involved in the signalling mechanism? *B J Hematol* , *120* (5), 829-839.

Lozoff, B. B. (2006). Long-Lasting Neural and Behavioral Effects of Iron Deficiency in Infancy. *Nutr Rev.* , 64(5 Pt 2): S34–S91.

Lukowski, A. K. (2010). Iron deficiency in infancy and neurocognitive functioning at 19 years: evidence of long-term deficits in executive function and recognition memory. *Nutr Neurosci* , *13* (2), 54-70.

Madan, N. R. (2010). Developmental and neurophysiologic deficits in iron deficient children. *Indian J Pediatr* , online.

Meena, A. N. (2000). Cortical sinovenous thrombosis in a child with nephrotic syndrome and iron deficiency anaemia. *Neurol India* , *48* (3), 292-4.

Micronutrient Information Centre. (n.d.). *Linus Pauling Institute*. (Linus Pauling Institute) Retrieved March 17, 2011, from http://lpi.oregonstate.edu/ infocenter/minerals/iron/ ironrefs.html#ref42

Mullick, S. R. (2006). Impact of iron deficiency anaemia on T lymphocytes and their subsets in children. *Indian J Med Res* , *124*, 647-654.

Murray, M. M. (1978). The Adverse Effect of Iron Repletion on the Course of Certain Infections. *Brit. Med J.* , *2*, 1113-1115.

Nemeth, E. R. (2004). IL-6 mediates hypoferremia of inflammation by inducing the synthesis of the iron regulatory hormone hepcidin. *J Clin Invest.* , *113* (9), 1251-3.

Park, C. V. (2001). Hepcidin, a Urinary Antimicrobial Peptide Synthesized in the Liver. *J Biol Chem* , *276*, 7806-10.

Pietrangelo, A. (2004). Non-HFE Hemochromatosis. *Hepatology* , *39* (1), 21-29.

Ready, W. L. (1989). Anemia causing cerebral infarction in a child. *CMAJ* , *140*, 303-304.

ReedGroup. (2011). *Anemia complicating Pregnancy*. Retrieved March 15, 2011, from MDGuidelines: http://www.mdguidelines.com/anemia-complicating-pregnancy

Rossi, E. (2005). Hepcidin - the iron regulatroy hormone. *Clin Biochem Rev* , *26*, 47-49.

Rushton, D. (2003). Decreased Serum Ferritin and Alopecia in Women. *J Inves Dermatol* , *121*, xvii–xviii.

Salmon, M. B. (1985). Transferrin receptor expression by stimulated cells in mixed lymphocyte culture. *Immunology* , *54*, 559.

Santos, P. F. (1990). Decreased lymphocyte subsets and K-cell activity in iron deficiency anemia. *Acta Haematol* , *84* (3), 118-21.

Schafer, A. (2004). N Engl J Med. *350*, 1211-121.

Sebire, G. T.-M. (2005). Cerebral venous sinus thrombosis in children: risk factors, presentation, diagnosis and outcome. *Brain* , *128*, 477-489.

Sébire, G. T.-M. (2005). Cerebral venous sinus thrombosis in children: risk factors, presentation, diagnosis and outcome. *Brain;128(Pt 3):* , *128* (Pt3), 477-89.

Stoltzfus, R. (2003). Iron deficiency: global prevalence and consequences. *Food Nutr Bull , 24* (4 Suppl), S99-103.

Stolz, E. V.-M. (2007). Anemia as a risk factor for cerebral venous thrombosis? An old hypothesis revisited. Results of a prospective study. *J Neurol , 254* (6), 729-34.

Weiss, G. G. (2005). Anemia of Chronic Disease. *N Engl J Med , 352* (10), 1011-1023.

Yager, J. B. (2008). Cerebral venous thrombosis in newborns, infants and children. *Front Neurol Neurosci , 23*, 122-31.

Yanoff, L. M. (2007). Inflammation and iron deficiency anemia in the hypoferremia of obesity. *International Journal of Obesity* , 31, 1412-1419.

Yeh, K. Y. (2009). Feeding induces ferroportin 1 and hephaestin migration and interaction duodenal epithelium. *Am J Physiol Gastrointest Liver Physiol , 296* , G55–G65.

Zhang, A. E. (2009). Iron Homeostasis: Recently identified proteins provide insight into novel control mechanisms. *Journal of Biological Chemistry , 284* (2), 711-715.

In: Iron Deficiency and Its Complications
Editor: Yildiz Dincer

ISBN 978-1-61324-854-6

Chapter 8

Short Bowel Syndrome and Anemia: Evidence beyond Iron Deficiency

Fabíola Rainato Gabriel*, Vivian Marques Miguel Suen, Julio Sergio Marchini and José Eduardo Dutra de Oliveira

Ribeirão Preto School of Medicine,
São Paulo University, Sao Paulo, Brazil

Abstract

Short bowel syndrome, as a consequence of extended small bowel resections, lead to nutritional deficiencies. Among them, iron deserves attention. Iron replacement therapy is a challenge due to intestinal malabsorption. In this scenario, the serum iron follow-up is recommended. The objective of the present study was to assess the course of serum iron, erythrocyte and biochemical iron markers up to 960 days after extended short bowel ressections. Erythrocyte and biochemical data from 37 enterectomized patients from the15th to the 960th post-surgery day were collected, adjusted and analyzed according to a random effect model. Forty-eight percent of the patients were found to have ferritin levels below normal limits and 78% had hemoglobin concentrations below normal limits. There was a gradual increase ($p<0.05$) in serum iron after enterectomy and changes in other erythrocytes indicators ($p <0.05$).

We conclude that although the malabsorption, short bowel syndrome patients showed increase in serum iron over time, probably due to intestinal adaptation mechanisms.

Keywords: short bowel syndrome, anemia, iron biochemical parameters, follow-up

* Corresponding author: Fabíola Rainato Gabriel, Division of Clinical Nutrition, Department of Internal Medicine, Hospital das Clinicas Ribeirão Preto School of Medicine, 6th Floor, Avenida dos Bandeirantes, 3900, Monte Alegre, Ribeirao Preto, Sao Paulo, Brazil. Zip Code: 14049-900. Phone: 55 16 3602 3375; Fax: 55 16 3633 6695, email: fabirainato@yahoo.com.br

Abbreviations

Unbinding iron binding capacity (UIBC)
Mmean corpuscular volume (VCM)
Mean corpuscular hemoglobin (HCM)
Mean corpuscular hemoglobin concentration (CHCM)

1. Introduction

Diseases of the digestive system that result in intestinal resections (enterectomy) lead to a reduced absorptive surface and a decreased intestinal transit time (< 15 minutes). The time of contact between the nutrients, the digestive secretions and the enterocytes decreases. This leads to malabsorption and malnutrition [1]. The general consequence is a clinical condition characterized by multiple nutrient deficiencies such as iron-deficiency anemia.

Iron-deficiency anemia is a nutritional problem commonly occurring in the hospital setting [2]. The physiopathological effects of iron deficiency may vary according to the stage of development and the rate of iron utilization of an individual. In general, iron deficiency occurs in a gradual and progressive manner, with three stages preceding the manifestation of the condition. The first stage is characterized by decreased iron stores and represents a period of greater vulnerability due to the marginal iron balance, eventually progressing to a more severe deficiency with functional consequences. The second stage is defined as iron-deficient erythropoiesis and is characterized by a lower than normal production of hemoglobin and other iron compounds even though the concentration of hemoglobin and of other iron compounds is not markedly reduced. The third and last stage is characterized by a reduction of hemoglobin levels. To our knowledge, studies investigating serum iron evolution in short bowel syndrome adults are scarce. Thus, the objective of the present study was to determine the erythrocyte and biochemical data related to iron metabolism follow-up in short bowel syndrome patients up to 960 days after intestinal resection.

2. Methods and Materials

Subjects

This study was previously approved by the Research Ethics Committee of the University Hospital, Faculty of Medicine of Ribeirão Preto, USP. The data were collectd from the medical records of all patients attended at Metabolic Unit from HCFMRP-USP.

Study Design

A survey of the number of patients who had undergone partial intestinal resection and who were monitored by the Clinical Nutrition Team at the Metabolic Unit Dutra de Oliveira

(UMDO), Department of Internal Medicine, was first performed. Then, the following data were collected for each patient, from the 15th to the 960th post-surgery day: date of birth, date of enterectomy, sex, etiology of surgery, intestinal portions resected, prescription of oral or intramuscular iron, erythrocyte parameters (erythrocytes, hemoglobin, hematocrit, mean corpuscular volume (MCV), hemoglobin, mean corpuscular hemoglobin (MCH), mean corpuscular hemoglobin concentration (MCHC) biochemical parameters (serum iron, unsaturated iron binding capacity (UIBC), serum ferritin) The data were tabulated and analyzed.

The present investigation did not interfere with the medical conduct to which the patients were submitted.

Statistical Analysis

Data were analyzed statistically using random effect models for longitudinal data [4] to calculate the mean levels of hemoglobin and of the other variables and their modifications along time. The MIXED procedure of the SAS computational software was used to adjust these models.

3. Results

A retrospective study was conducted on 37 enterectomized subjects (19 females, 51%, and 18 males, 49%) ranging in age from 25 to 83 years (mean age: 51±15 years).

The underlying disorders that caused the short bowel syndrome were: mesenteric ischemia (70%), intestinal twisting (6%) intestinal occlusion (8%), perforated duodenal ulcer (6%) and acute appendicitis and cecum perforation (3%), unknown (5%). The remaining gut was composed of duodenum and half jejunum. One hundred percent of the patients did not have remaining ileum and ileocecal valve.

Mean ferritin levels were not considered since this exam was seldom requested. However, it should be pointed out that practically half the subjects studied (48.6%) tended to have lower ferritin levels after surgery. Mean serum iron levels after surgery were about 50 µg/dL, followed by a significant progressive increase (Logtime, $p = 0.019$), with no difference between sexes. Iron binding capacity did not differ significantly between sexes during follow-up and was within normal limits throughout the study.

Mean erythrocyte values were below normal levels in both sexes and continued to be below normal throughout follow-up. Hemoglobin values were below normal levels in 78% of cases, indicating an extremely high incidence of anemia throughout patient follow-up. Hematocrit values decreased in a progressive and significant manner ($p < 0.05$) during the first 60 days after surgery and increased gradually after this period. MCV did not differ between sexes or during follow-up. MCH was within lower normal limits or below normal but did not differ during the study period. MCHC also decreased during the follow-up period and differed significantly between sexes and throughout the study period ($p < 0.05$) (Table 1 and Table 2).

Table 1. Hematologic paramenters from admission to 960 days after small bowel resection for female sex

	Admission	15	30	60	120	240	480	960	> 960
UIBC (ug/dL)	229	230	231	231	231	232	232	232	233
Red cell (10^6/Ul)	3.4	3.6	3.6	3.7	3.7	3.8	3.8	3.8	3.9
Hemoglobin (g/dL)	10	11	10.6	10.7	10.8	10.9	11	11	11
Hematocrite (%)	36	31	31	31.5	32.2	33	34	34.6	35
VCM (fL)	78	84	85.8	87	87.9	88.5	89	88.8	88
HCM (Pg)	2	28	28.6	29	29.3	29.4	29	29.2	27
CHCM (g/dL)	34	32	30.9	30.3	29.6	28.9	28	27.6	26

UIBC = unbinding iron binding capacity, VCM = mean corpuscular volume, HCM = mean corpuscular hemoglobin, CHCM = mean corpuscular hemoglobin concentration.

Table 2. Hematologic paramenters from admission to 960 days after small bowel resection for male sex

	Admission	15	30	60	120	240	480	960	> 960
UIBC (ug/Dl)	213	215	215	215	216	216	216	217	218
Red cell (10^6/Ul)	3.3	3.5	3.5	3.6	3.6	3.7	2.7	3.7	3.8
Hemoglobin (g/dL)	11	10,9	11	11	11	11	11.4	11.5	11.5
Hematocrite (%)	36	31	31	31.5	32.3	33	33.9	34.7	35.2
VCM (fL)	81	85.8	88.3	89.5	90.5	91	91.3	91.3	91
HCM (Pg)	27	28.6	30.5	30.8	31	31	31.2	31	29,5
CHCM (g/dL)	35	30.9	31.9	31.2	30.6	30	29.3	28.6	26.5

UIBC = unbinding iron binding capacity, VCM = mean corpuscular volume, HCM = mean corpuscular hemoglobin, CHCM = mean corpuscular hemoglobin concentration.

The frequency of prescription of iron supplementation was about 75.7%. The route most used for iron administration was the exclusively intramuscular one (35%), while the exclusively oral route was the least used (11%).

4. Discussion

To our knowledge, few studies regarding longitudinal follow-up of iron-deficiency anemia in individuals with short bowel syndrome have been published.

In the present study were observed that patients with short bowel syndrome presented changes in the biochemical iron indicators. The frequency of hemoglobin values below normal limits throughout the follow-up period indicated an extremely high and persistent prevalence of anemia after intestinal surgery according to the criteria of the World Health Organization [5].

In a randomized study, Mei et al. (2005) [6] showed that ferritin and hemoglobin represent the most efficient combination for the monitoring of changes in iron status in the population. The results of the present study suggest that our patients had iron-deficiency anemia at several time points after surgery due to their lower than normal values of both ferritin and hemoglobin.

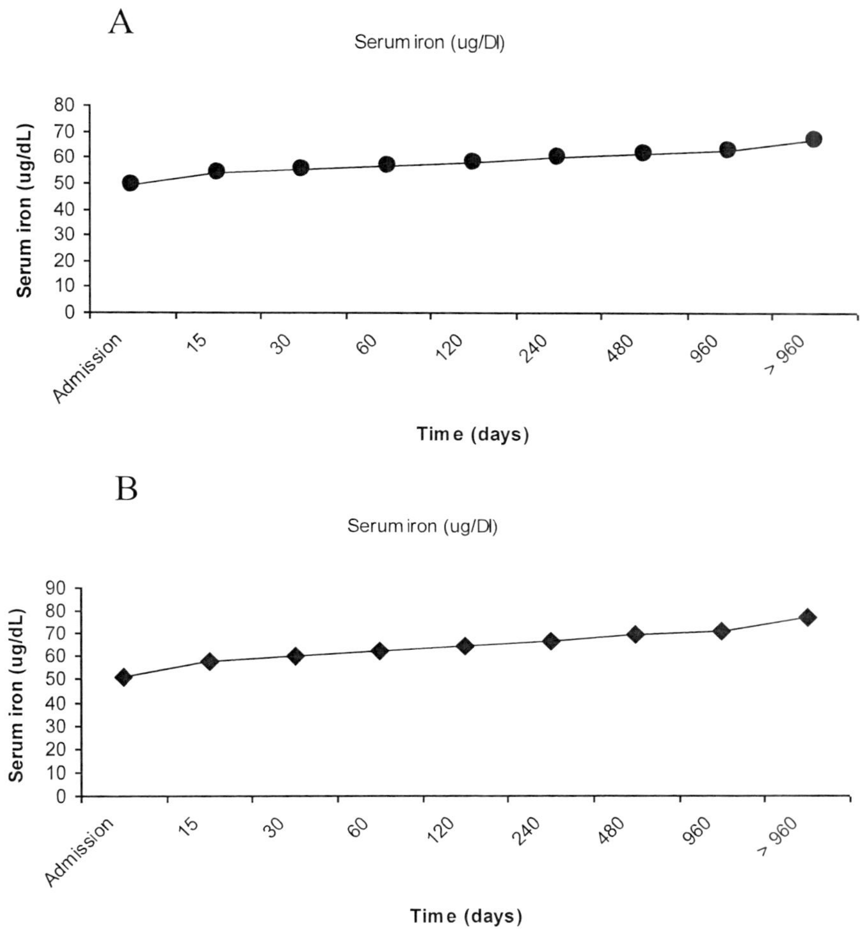

Figure 1. Serum iron levels from admission to more than 960 days after enterectomy. A = Male; B = Female.

It should be pointed out that ferritin is an acute phase protein that may be normal or elevated in inflammatory or neoplastic diseases but does not expresses correctly the amount of stored iron [7]. Some enterectomized patients tended to have higher ferritin levels, a fact that may be due to inflammatory or neoplastic diseases or to iron accumulation. However it was not the objective of the present study to characterize other abnormalities of iron metabolism in addition to iron deficiency. In a retrospective study [8] the amount of stored iron was correlated with serum ferritin and the authors observed that about 50% of the patients with absence of medullary iron presented normal serum ferritin levels and one third of the patients with iron deficiency presented ferritin levels higher than 100 μg/dL. Thus, patients with high ferritin levels may also present iron deficiency. With the reduction of stored iron there will also be a reduction of circulating iron and an increase in iron binding capacity to transferrin in plasma [9,10]. We may state that most of the serum iron and UIBC values measured after surgery were within normal limits according to the reference values adopted (35-150 μg/dL and 112-346 μg/dL, respectively).

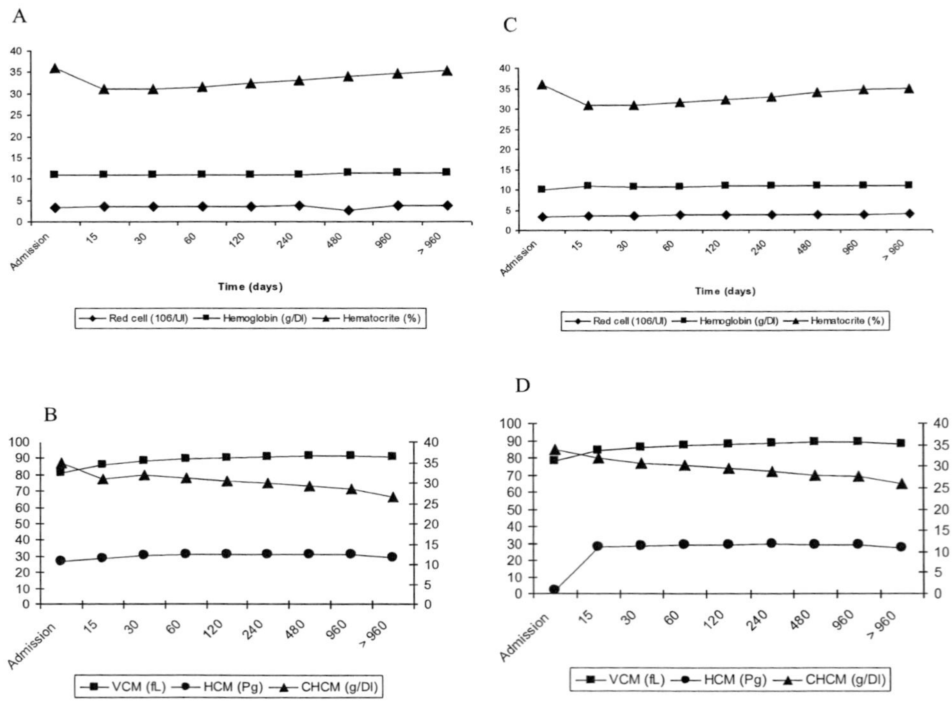

Figure 2. Evolution of hematologic values from admission to more than 960 days after surgery. A and B = Male; C and D = Female.

Serum iron levels were often about 50 μg/dL, with a gradual increase over time ($p < 0.05$). UIBC did not change significantly. The limitation of the present study is that iron concentration may also change in the presence of infectious processes, possibly decreasing within a few hours after the triggering of an infection. Total UIBC increases in iron deficiency but decreases in the presence of inflammation, thus providing evidence for differentiation between the two situations. However, it should be evaluated in a judicious manner since it may be within the normal range when both inflammation and iron deficiency are present [10]. Thus, ferritin, serum iron and UIBC may be within normal limits in patients with short bowel syndrome and, due to some limitations of these indices, they may mask the real situation of iron status.

Hepcidin, a 25-amino acid peptide exclusively synthesized by the liver, is acknowledged to be an iron regulatory hormone. The synthesis and release of hepcidin is rapidly mediated by cytokine release. The increased hepcidin release leads to decreased iron absorption by the enterocytes. Cytokine mediated induction of hepcidin caused by inflammation is now thought to be responsible for the anaemia of chronic disease, low transferrin saturation, iron-restricted erythropoeisis and mild to moderate anemia. Short bowel syndrome has been shown to be accompanied by an inflammatory state which might contribute to anemia. [11,12,13].

We conclude that although the malabsorption, short bowel syndrome patients showed increase in serum iron over time, probably due to intestinal adaptation mechanisms. Further studies are needed regarding the intestinal role in iron metabolism in short bowel syndrome.

Acknowledgment

We are thankful to CNPq for funding the research.

References

[1] Navarro AM, Suen VM, Souza IM, De Oliveira JE, Marchini JS. Patients with severe bowel malabsorption do not have changes in iodine status. *Nutrition* 2005; 21: 895-900.

[2] Waitzberg DL, Caiaffa WT, Correia MI. Hospital malnutrition: the Brazilian national survey (IBRANUTRI): a study of 4000 patients. *Nutrition* 2001; 17: 573-80.

[3] Laird NM, Ware JH. Random effect models for longitudinal data. *Biometrics* 1982; 38: 963-74.

[4] Linker CA. Blood disorders. In: McPhee SJ, Papadakis MA. *Current Medical Diagnosis and Treatment.* New York: Mc Graw Hill; 2008. p. 422-24.

[5] WORLD HEALTH ORGANIZATION. Iron deficiency anaemia. Assessment, prevention, and control. A guide for programmed managers Commission on Health and Environment. *Report of the panel on food and agriculture*. Geneva, 2001.

[6] Mei Z, Cogswell Me, Parvanta I, Lynch S, Beard Jl, Stoltzfus Rj, Grummer-Strawn Lm. Hemoglobin and ferritin are currently the most efficient indicators of population response to iron interventions: an analysis of nine randomized controlled trials. *J Nutr* 2005; 135: 1974-80.

[7] Brugnara, C. Iron deficiency and erythropoiesis: new diagnostic approaches. *Clinical Chemistry* 2003; 49: 1573-78.

[8] Birgegard G, Hallgren R, Killander A, Stromberg A, Venge P, Wide L. Serum Ferritin during infection. *A longitudinal study. Scandinavian Journal of Hematology* 1978; 21: 333-340.

[9] Stengle JM, Shade AL. Diurnal-nocturnal variations of certain blood constituents in normal human subjects: plasma iron, siderophilin, bilirubin, copper, total serum protein and albumin, haemoglobin and hematocrit. *British Journal of Haematology* 1957; 3: 117-122.

[10] Cook JD. Diagnosis and management of iron-deficiency anaemia. *Best Practice Research Clinical Haematology* 2005; 18: 319-332.

[11] Compher C, Pazianas M, Benedic S, Brown JC, Kinosian BP, Hise, M. Systemic Inflammatory mediators and bone homeostasis in intestinal failure. Journal of Parenteral and Enteral Nutrition 2007; 31:142-7.

[12] Nemeth E, Ganz T. Regulation of iron metabolism by hepcidin. *Ann Rev Nutr* 2006; 26: 323-42.

[13] Piperno A, Mariani R, Trombini P, Girelli D. Hepcidin modulation in human diseases: from research to clinic. *World* J. Gastroenterol 2009; 15: 538-51.

Index

C

D

E

F

G

H

I

J

K

L

M

N

O

P

Q

R

S

T

U

V

W

X

Y

Z